BLACK NOTLEY BLUES

To Gan
with best wishes.

Colins   18⁴/₉

BLACK NOTLEY BLUES

Diary of a teenage TB patient
1958—1959

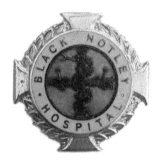

CHRIS DELL

London

BLACK NOTLEY BLUES

Hardback 978-0-9926785-1-7
Paperback 978-0-9926785-0-0

First published in Great Britain in 2013 by Stortford Documentation Services,
Bishops Stortford, Hertfordshire CM23 3JW

British Library Cataloguing in Publication Data.
A CIP catalogue record for this book is available from the British Library.

The author and publisher has made all reasonable efforts to contact copyright
holders for permissions, and apologises for any omissions or errors in the form
of credits given. Corrections may be made to future printings.

The following photographs have been reproduced with permission of
Braintree District Museum Trust Ltd: the aerial photograph of Black Notley
Hospital (Cover, p. xiv), the photograph of Mr Michael Wilkinson (p. 4)
and the Black Notley Hospital main entrance (p. 9),
www.braintreemuseum.co.uk.

Typeset in 11pt Electra by Abstract Graphics, Herts

Printed and bound in
Great Britain by Lightning Source UK Ltd,
Milton Keynes MK11 3LW

To my wife Carole,
for her encouragement
and to all former staff and patients
during my time at Black Notley Hospital,
wherever they may be.

CONTENTS

FOREWORD VIII

PREFACE X

PART 1
BLACK NOTLEY BLUES 1

PART 2
THE ROAD TO RECOVERY 95

PART 3
RETURN VISITS 115

ACKNOWLEDGEMENTS 123

Foreword

When the new, purpose built tuberculosis sanatorium at Black Notley was opened on 26 April 1930, there were in Britain 420 TB institutions caring for 26,500 patients. About eight people in every 10,000 died of TB, and the highest death rates were among the young productive members of society, particularly the age group fifteen to twenty-five. Those who survived were often left with chronic lung disease or were physically disabled. Many were unable to work or were denied work because of the stigma of being labelled 'tubercular'.

The real breakthrough in the treatment of TB came in the 1940s with the discovery of streptomycin, the world's second antibiotic (the first was penicillin), and the development of adjuvant drugs over the next decade. These worked by killing or inhibiting growth of the bacteria which caused TB. By the time Chris Dell was admitted to Black Notley Hospital in 1958, the atmosphere in most TB sanatoria was more relaxed and positive than in previous decades because effective drug treatment not only offered hope of a cure but also made possible the complex orthopaedic procedures undergone by Chris and his ward mates.

There are less than a handful of personal testimonies detailing life in a tuberculosis sanatorium, and this is the first daily diary I have ever seen. As a record of institutional humdrum, it is a surprisingly entertaining read; throw in 'Boy's Own' camaraderie, nurse-chasing, illicit pub crawls and regular carpeting by Matron and Medical Superintendent, and it has all the ingredients of a 'Carry On' comedy. Yet beneath the fun and games this is an important medical, social and personal record of the 1950s sanatorium experience where occupational therapy, operations, pain, plaster boats, courage, rehabilitation and daily Guinness meet Grundig tape recorders, chess matches, pen pals, bats, Beethoven and Buddy Holly.

A physician who worked in the 1950s once told me that *'TB males were difficult to control in the days of a strict regimen.'* This is typical of the doctor-centred accounts of medicine that go down in history as 'truth'. Chris Dell's diary offers an important alternative perspective, that of the patient – in this case a mischievous, courageous teenager who 'brought a ray of sunshine' to Black Notley Hospital.

DR CAROLE REEVES

Senior Lecturer in Science and Technology Studies
UCL Science and Technology Studies
University College London

PREFACE

The first part of the book covers my time as a 19 year old patient at Black Notley Hospital from 12 August 1958 until 19 May 1959. The second part covers my convalescence at the Caxton Memorial Home in Deal and further recovery in the Essex countryside and Scandinavia. The third part concludes with re-visits, recent photographs and Acknowledgements paying tribute to my family and friends who supported me during this difficult time.

My stay at Black Notley spanned a period of 280 days which might sound an eternity but many other patients, especially from earlier years, were confined for very much longer – in some cases over several years, and some very young children were adolescent by the time of discharge.

My experiences described here are supported by primary source evidence from daily diary entries, photographs, letters to friends and my own memory of people, places and events.

I have not typed up the diary entries word for word because the small space available for each day sometimes required my own shorthand and abbreviations to record each event. In any case, much of the text was written while laying flat on my back thereby making neatness something of a rarity.

The events are reported exactly as occurred with nothing added, although I have applied just a little censoring here and there. In a few instances I have used an alias for certain individuals to protect their identity.

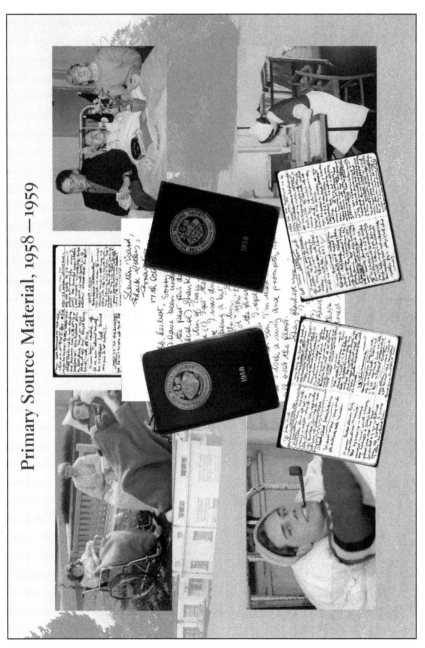

Primary Source Material, 1958—1959

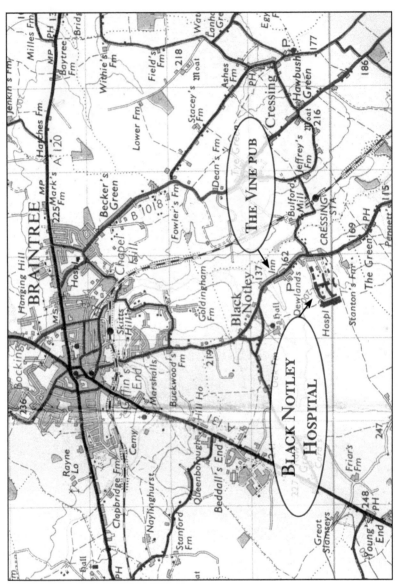

Map of the Braintree district showing the hospital complex
before development into housing in 1998.
Map: © Crown Copyright 1957.

Black Notley Hospital was opened in 1900 equipped with just eight beds and a horse-drawn ambulance. The purpose was to isolate and treat patients suffering from contagious diseases such as smallpox, diphtheria, scarlet fever, cholera, typhoid and tuberculosis. In 1912 plans were prepared to extend the facility into a sanatorium which opened in 1930 with 160 beds increasing to 300 by 1937.

The next decade saw the hospital expanded to include 19 wards, an operating theatre, an x-ray department, a nurses' home and other facilities spread over 20 acres. The theatre had three operating tables allowing simultaneous operations to be carried out in the same room.

During World War II the hospital treated casualties from air raids, foreign refugees, evacuees, civil defence workers and military personnel from the international fighting services.

By the early 1960s the incidence of tuberculosis more or less ceased so the sanatorium wards were used to treat other conditions such as cerebral palsy and orthopaedic work. In the 1990s the hospital began to be phased out when patients and staff were transferred to Broomfield and Colchester hospitals. In 1998 and after a century of honourable service, Black Notley Hospital finally surrendered to a housing estate while retaining its delightful open areas of lawns and trees.

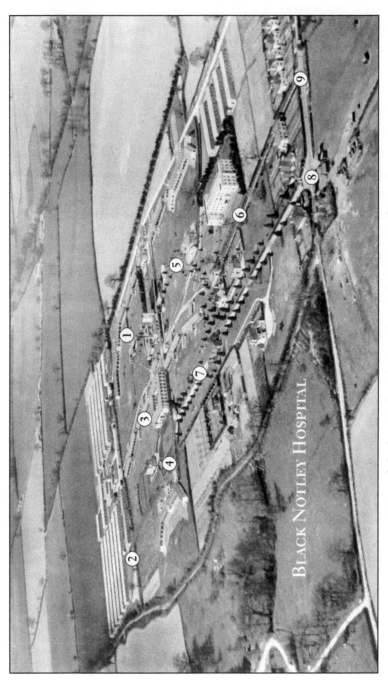

View of the hospital with the relevant buildings indicated.
Photo: Courtesy of Braintree District Museum Trust Ltd.

① Ward 8
Stayed in Ward 8 from 12 August 1958 to 30 September 1958

② Denton Ward and Astins Ward run parallel in this block.
Stayed in Denton Ward from 30 September 1958 to 21 April 1959

③ Ward 1
Stayed in Ward 1 from 21 April 1959 to 18 May 1959

④ Catholic Church

⑤ Canteen and Social Centre

⑥ Nurses' Home

⑦ Memorial Hall

⑧ Main Entrance

⑨ To The Vine Pub

PART 1

BLACK NOTLEY BLUES

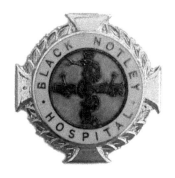

PART 1

BLACK NOTLEY BLUES

Tuesday 12 August 1958

My friend Alan McEwan came round to my home at 25 Putney Road, Enfield and joined Pop, Mum and sister Susan (Ginger) in the car taking me to Black Notley Hospital near Braintree. I was put to bed in a single room on Ward 8. Doors and windows were left open and the front exposed to the chilly night air. Forbidden to get up – bed pans, bottles and boredom, ah well, that's life. Another patient came in with a chess set and I lost – not a good start. Italian male orderlies Joe and Tony are on night duty.

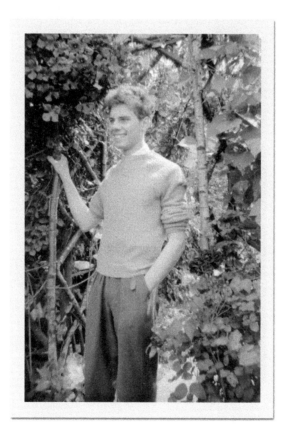

Aged 19 in my back garden, the day before admission.
Don't know what I'm smiling about!

I lay gazing at the ceiling wondering what the hell I am doing here. The answer is simple, my own silly fault; the architect of my own misfortune. Three months in Napier Ward, Chase Farm Hospital in 1955 put me off hospitals – wanted no more of it. So when I started feeling poorly again I took analgesics hoping the problem would go away but it didn't and I had to surrender to the inevitable. But now I'm here I'll make the best of this new adventure – just a bloody nuisance that's all.

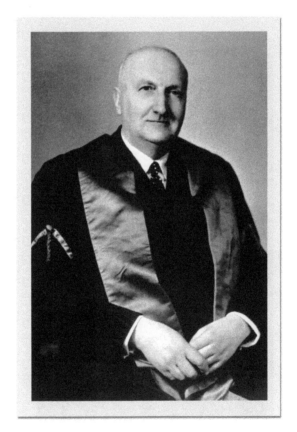

Mr Michael Wilkinson,
Medical Superintendent and Orthopaedic Surgeon.
Photo: Courtesy of Braintree District Museum Trust Ltd.

Wednesday 13 August 1958

Had the first of a weekly blood test then the orderlies shoved me outside into more fresh air. Head Surgeon Mr Michael Wilkinson (known as Wilkie) and another doctor arrived and pushed me through the corridor, I later named *Bed Pan Alley*, into the day room and laid me on a dining table. Wilkie examined me by pulling me around which really hurt so I punched him on the arm to make him stop – he was rather amused by that. They put me back to bed and wrapped me in a straightjacket, elastic stockings, splints and traction, and a metal frame over me to take the weight of the blankets. I feel just like an oven-ready chicken. The mattress is hard and to make it worse they put planks of wood underneath which made it feel like I am lying on a bed of concrete. During the night some bats flew into my room and sat on the metal frame staring at me. Nice to have a bit of company I suppose. I half expected Christopher Lee to appear with bared fangs. I wish I had brought my crucifix or some garlic!

Thursday 14 August 1958

Quite comfortable now – getting used to the splints. Had the first of my daily injection of streptomycin, it's meant to kill off the nasty little bugs invading my body.

Friday 15 August 1958

Doctor gave me some morphine. Should have kept quiet about the pain because I spewed up all day. Rather suffer than go hungry so I tried to reject the next dose but they gave it to me anyway. Makes me sick every time – allergic?

Saturday 16 August 1958

Eaten nothing since Thursday but settling down. Bit bored really – not used to lying in bed all day and night. Prefer to be out playing or down my local pub in Enfield, the Prince Albert with my mates.

Sunday 17 August 1958

Brother Brian and Alan visited me – pleased to see them.

Monday 18 August 1958

Feeling much better and eating again. Letters arrived from the staff of Halifax Building Society (HBS) where I work. The Society agreed to pay my full wages for six months then half wages until I return to work – very good of them. Other patients popped into my room to say hello including footballer Bill Simmons. They told me that singer Tommy Steele had arrived by helicopter a while ago and landed on the grass outside to entertain the patients. Don't know if they were pulling my leg – I'll leave that to the traction. Anyway it's a pity I missed him 'singing the blues'.

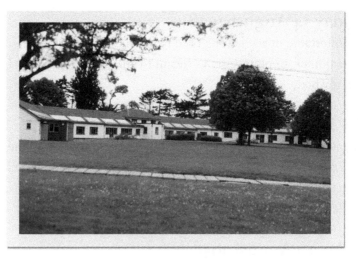

If this is not Ward 8, it is another ward very similar.

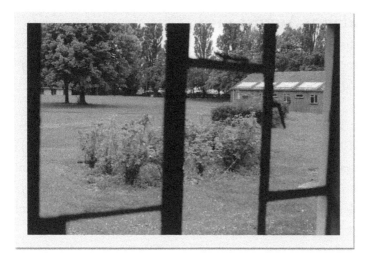

This is the view through the window of my room on Ward 8.
Normally the doors and windows were open all the time. As it's
day time I reckon my bats were roosting in the trees opposite.

Tuesday 19 August 1958

Had more injections and feel fine today. Cards from Ivor Snowden and
John Allen, still at Tottenham County School. Had my first bed bath
and daily ration of Guinness. It must be good for you as the toucan
says. Not much to complain about but I wish there were some female
nurses instead of the male Italians. Maybe they don't trust the long-term
patients – maybe they have a good reason.

Wednesday 20 August 1958

Letter from HBS manager Harry Greenwood. Parcel of books from
Miss Violet Phinn – a retired maths teacher from Tottenham County
School living at the top of Putney Road where I live. One of the cushions
was removed from under my legs. Still nightly visits from the bats.

Thursday 21 August 1958

Had my first hospital hair cut from the visiting barber. Letters arrived from school friends Joe Trow and Doreen Picking, and others from the HBS staff.

Friday 22 August 1958

Alan McEwan came to see me during the afternoon – he hitch-hiked to the hospital. Evening, listened to the proms on the wireless earphones – Beethoven's *Leonora no. 1*, *Piano Concerto no. 3* and *Symphony no. 2*. It reminded me of the fun we had with the Cooperative Youth Orchestra last May with me on the double bass.

Saturday 23 August 1958

Down to one cushion now. Letters arrived from Doreen Price and the HBS staff. I dropped and broke my daily ration of Guinness. They wouldn't give me another one.

Sunday 24 August 1958

Mum, Pop, John and Alan visited me in the afternoon. John is now working for Allen & Hanbury's in Ware, and Alan is soon going to Hull University as a student. John brought my Grundig tape recorder which is great. Another patient, Harry Green, doesn't like Guinness so we made a deal; he gives me his daily ration in exchange for me rolling his tobacco to make fags. His arm is in a sling and he cannot do it himself. I will now get two bottles of Guinness a day – things are looking up. Perhaps I'll get better twice as fast.

Monday 25 August 1958

John and Alan McEwan came in the afternoon – they bummed a lift to get here. Really great to see them. Doctors did their rounds afterwards. Wilkie introduced Dr Brahma, his assistant.

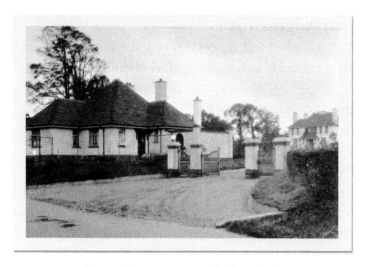

The main entrance to the hospital.
Photo: Courtesy of Braintree District Museum Trust Ltd.

Tuesday 26 August 1958

Letters arrived from Joe and Doreen, and others from the HBS. Still on my own in a single room with the bats every night – maybe they will move me in with other patients for some human company. I don't mind the bats as long as they don't make a mess on my bed.

Wednesday 27 August 1958

Nice card from Mrs Phipps (Ann Cawthorne's mother) from Hoddesdon – must write back. Not much else going on. Started making a teddy bear from stuff provided by Occupational Therapy (OT).

Thursday 28 August 1958

They put me back to four cushions again – not very comfortable.

Friday 29 August 1958

More letters arrived – I will answer them all. Joe and Doreen said they were coming but didn't turn up. Shaved for nothing.

Saturday 30 August 1958

Not much doing today – very quiet.

Sunday 31 August 1958

Wilkie back today. Brothers Brian and Ron visited me in the afternoon. At last I was moved to a room with four beds occupied by Bill Webb, Bill (Stubby) Lagdon and one empty bed. Played chess with Stubby across the ward by calling out the coordinates. He usually wins.

Monday 1 September 1958

Things are looking up – a fine young lady doctor came round with Wilkie and examined me in the day room. He told me I am the only male patient in the hospital with my condition so I must expect a lot of visits from the medical staff, internal and external.

Tuesday 2 September 1958

Another quiet day, nothing much to report.

Wednesday 3 September 1958

Finished working on the teddy bear. Saw some fine women out the front of the ward. Don't get any working here.

Thursday 4 September 1958

Went down for an x-ray. Had a laugh with the radiologist but she said I was cheeky and threatened to send me straight back to the ward without doing the x-ray if I didn't behave. So I behaved and she took the x-ray.

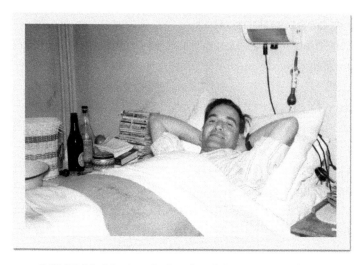

*Bill Webb. Notice the bottle of Guinness and one
of the baskets that we made from cane.*

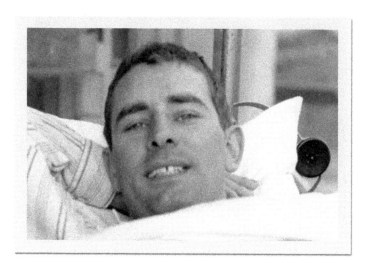

*Another cell-mate and my chess opponent
Bill (Stubby) Lagdon from Dagenham, Essex.*

Friday 5 September 1958

Mr and Mrs Trow, Joe and Doreen came to see me in the evening.
Biggest storm and lightning of the century.

Saturday 6 September 1958

Quiet day – not much to report.

Sunday 7 September 1958

Mum, Pop, Susan (Ginger) and Ron visited me. Brought Tex our dog
with them – great to see them all, especially Tex. They brought my
microphone for the Grundig. Now that I have the microphone, I can
record stuff. For a start I recorded Staff Nurse Taffy Price singing Welsh
folk songs. Bloody awful but entertaining.

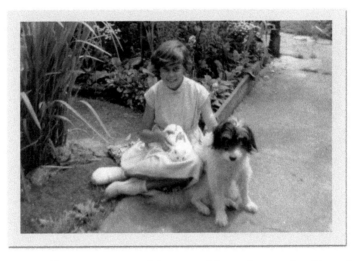

*My sister Ginger came to visit me and brought our dog Tex, who
was allowed on the ward. Billy the rabbit had to stay at home.*

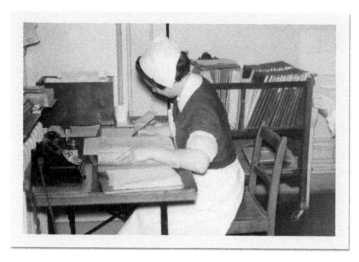

Sister Kathleen Bartholomew – I became the bane of her life,
the pain in her neck. That's what she told me anyway.

Monday 8 September 1958

Wilkie did his rounds. I spent the day knitting a yellow sweater for Alan
with a cello on the back. Designed my own pattern.

Tuesday 9 September 1958

Not a lot going on today. Started making cane baskets with materials
from OT by first soaking the canes in a bowl of water to soften them up.

Wednesday 10 September 1958

Borrowed Bill Webb's record player and recorded some music onto the
Grundig. Gives me something else to do and keeps me out the pubs –
wishful thinking.

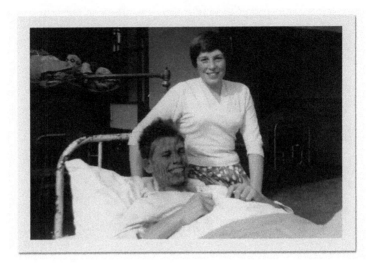

Me with Ann Cawthorne. Don't know who blacked my face.
Perhaps I was to audition for the Black and White Minstrels show.

Thursday 11 September 1958
New boy Ray from Buntingford moved into the ward. Two patients from
another room got an early discharge because they came in drunk last
night – let that be a warning.

Friday 12 September 1958
Finished the back of Alan's sweater. Recorded Mozart's *K 491 Piano*
Concerto from the wireless. Special permit to have my bed moved to the
day room so I can watch tele.

Saturday 13 September 1958
Bit of a panic on the ward as Bill Webb was stung in the mouth by a
wasp hiding in his fruit drink. Sister Kathleen Bartholomew sorted him
out and Orderly Joe sorted out the wasp.

Sunday 14 September 1958

Brother Brian and Ann Cawthorne came to see me on the back of his motorbike. He has owned several motorbikes including a 1934 Royal Enfield, a 500cc 1938 Rudge Special and a 1000cc 1952 Arial Square 4 with sidecar.

Monday 15 September 1958

Saw Wilkie in the day room. He said I am doing OK but will need surgery later on. Recorded Tchaikovsky's *Pathetique Symphony*. That didn't do much to cheer me up.

Tuesday 16 September 1958

Not a lot doing. Continued knitting Alan's yellow sweater. Started on the sleeves now – left the tricky bits till last.

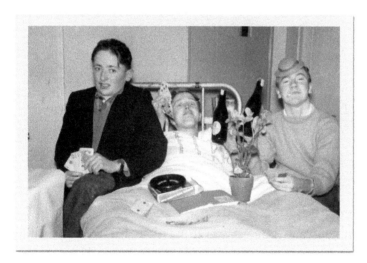

Hughie Keating (left) with his mates playing cards and roulette.
He has a spinal problem and cannot turn his head in either direction.

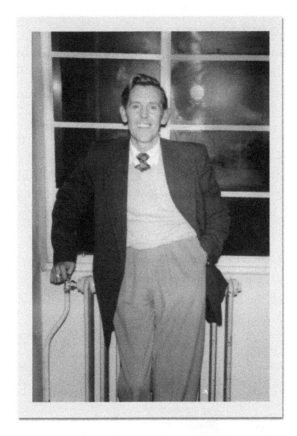

*Len West – has a severe curvature in his spine propped
up by a rib. He came to my home after demob.*

Wednesday 17 September 1958

Afternoon, John and Alan visited me. Could only stay for half an hour
because of a dental appointment. Evening, had a good laugh with
patients Len West, Hughie Keating, Ron, Stubby and Bill in a recording
session on my Grundig – chatting, singing, telling jokes.

Thursday 18 September 1958

For something to do I suggested that we could write a play using the patients as actors and record it. I got to work on the script and called it *Black Notley Blues*. It was about a new patient Mr Neverjabbed being admitted for an ingrowing toenail but he ended up spending several months in the hospital. For the hospital staff, Mr Wilkinson became Mr Winkleson, Dr Brahma became Dr Drama, and Sister Bartholomew became Sister Bathcube etc.

Friday 19 September 1958

Recorded Vaughan-Williams *Fantasia on a Theme of Thomas Tallis* and Beethoven's *Symphony no. 7* from the wireless. Finished writing the script for our play and copied it for rehearsal tomorrow. Gave my script to a nurse who took it home for typing up and copying.

Saturday 20 September 1958

Day to rehearse the play. Stubby, Bill Webb, Bill Simmons, Ron, Len, Ray, Jock, Hughie and I were the actors. Had to use my hand-written parts until they were typed up and copied. Made a test recording on the Grundig to see how it came out. Evening, went to the day room to watch *Cheyenne* on the tele.

Sunday 21 September 1958

Mum, Pop and Miss Violet Phinn visited me. Sold her one of my hand-made baskets for 15 bob. I think she wanted it for nothing but I need the cash to buy materials from OT for the next basket.

Monday 22 September 1958

Wilkie did his rounds. Quiet day. Busted my wristwatch. Asked an orderly if he would take it to the menders.

Tuesday 23 September 1958
Went down for an x-ray. Radiologist reminded me not to be cheeky. Me cheeky? Perish the thought.

Wednesday 24 September 1958
John, Alan and SAJ Brown visited me in the afternoon. Alan and SAJ are going to Hull University. Recorded Beethoven's *Symphony no. 3* and Mendelssohn's *Fingal's Cave* from Hughie's wireless earphones.

Thursday 25 September 1958
Got my watch back – cost 9 bob. Nothing exciting today except a young female doctor waved as she passed the ward. She wore a white coat so must have been a doctor, or maybe a painter and decorator. I think she fancies me.

Friday 26 September 1958
Another quiet day – not much happening.

Saturday 27 September 1958
Recorded from the wireless Tchaikovsky's *Romeo and Juliet* and Brahms' *Tragic Overture*.

Sunday 28 September 1958
Brian and Uncle Eddie arrived on a motor bike.

Monday 29 September 1958
Chinese doctor came with Wilkie on his rounds. Recorded some of the patients singing – bloody awful.

Tuesday 30 September 1958
Moved us all from Ward 8 to Denton Ward – I was last to go. They want to decorate Ward 8. Letter from Joe Trow.

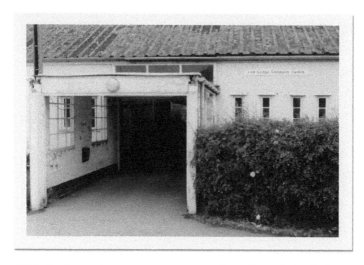

*This is the main entrance to a number of wards including
Denton Ward, where we moved to, and Astins Ward
for children and teenagers.*

Wednesday 1 October 1958

Nearly finished Alan's sweater. Ken Lovett was chatting up girls in
the adjacent Astins Ward across the grass. They won't catch me doing
that – fraternising with nurses and female patients is forbidden. Wilkie
came and said he will cut me up on 14 October. Something not to
look forward to.

Thursday 2 October 1958

Wilkie came to see me in the morning to tell me there is little hope of a
full recovery. Never mind, it's my silly fault I'm here so I can't complain.
Clifford Glascoe, branch manager of the Halifax Building Society (HBS)
in Braintree, visited in afternoon. Nice chap, stayed for two hours.

Friday 3 October 1958

Quiet day – finished another basket. Getting good at this lark and hope
to make some serious money.

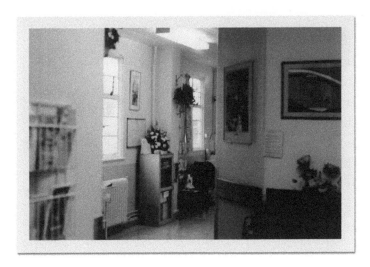

Entrance to Denton Ward itself. Denton Ward and Astins Ward run parallel to each other about 20 feet apart separated by a grass verge. Patients and staff from each ward could see each other through the doors and windows across the divide.

Saturday 4 October 1958

Another quiet day apart from us all listening again to our play rehearsal on the tape recorder. Always cheers us up.

Sunday 5 October 1958

Pop, Mum, Alan and Maureen Copsey visited me in the afternoon. Then I recorded Beethoven's *Waldstein Sonata*.

Monday 6 October 1958

Wilkie saw me in the day room with a crowd of fine young student nurses and Sister. Wilkie is using my case for a lecture to junior surgeons. I feel important now!

Tuesday 7 October 1958

Tried to see Sister for information about the operation but she was too busy. Stubby starts his treatment today but Ray is getting on our nerves with his chattering. If he doesn't shut up I'll chuck a bed pan at him, preferably full.

Wednesday 8 October 1958

Clifford Glascoe came to see me and to ask about the operation. I told him I'm not too worried about the surgery, only the possible outcome – will I get back to normal (whatever that is) or not? But sod it, let's be optimistic – of course I'll be OK. Wilkie is the best.

Thursday 9 October 1958

Started a new basket, doing good business flogging them.

Friday 10 October 1958

Dr. Brahma gave me two jabs then Staff Nurses George Moase and Taffy Price changed the traction weights. I will need at least two pints of blood during the operation. Hope it's good stuff.

Saturday 11 October 1958

Bit of a barney going on in the ward. Ken Lovett and others were accused of fraternising with the female nurses. Strictly forbidden according to Deputy Matron Miss Palmer. Shame on them – she won't catch me doing that.

Sunday 12 October 1958

Sister on holiday. Mum, Pop and Tug Wilson visited and saw Wilkie and Dr Brahma about the operation. Orderlies moved me to a single room ready for the op.

Monday 13 October 1958

The local vicar came in to see me – bloody hell it's not that serious is it? Glad he didn't give me the last rights. Staff Nurse George prepared me for theatre. They told me the operation is called a debridement. Getting a bit nervous now – especially with that Catholic vicar turning up. I am Church of England and told him so. If he hadn't shown up I would have felt better but I'm sure he meant well. I'm bound to be here tomorrow to continue my diary.

Tuesday 14 October 1958

Staff Nurse Taffy painted me with iodine and gave me a pre-med injection to make me relaxed and sleepy but my ear was buzzing like mad. Domestic Ron Haylock pushed me across the cold grounds to the operating theatre. Two fine young nurses there – that's the last thing I remember. Next thing I recall was me yelling for water.

Wednesday 15 October 1958.

Pop phoned the hospital to see how I was. Haven't eaten since before the operation. Spewed and spewed all day. The morphine injections made me feel worse.

Thursday 16 October 1958

Still eating nothing but feeling a bit better. Taffy changed the bandages – have a fine scar to show off now. A load more weights hanging from me – don't like it. Feel like I'm being stretched on a rack like in those Hammer horror films with Vincent Price.

Friday 17 October 1958

Wilkie came in to see me. Still not eating much. Orderly Mrs Harris gave me some foul stuff to clear me out. She's a middle-aged woman who takes no nonsense from anyone, especially me. Listened to *Symphonie Fantastique* by Berlioz. Wrote to Alan at his digs at Hull

University who enrolled a week or so ago, thanking him for the tin of Bass that arrived just before my operation. I told him I drank the Bass after my pre-med injection and was violently sick on the bed. Mrs Harris warned not to do it, but did I listen?

Saturday 18 October 1958

Feeling much better today – Mrs Harris's evil potion did the trick. Lots of activity along Bed Pan Alley. Taken back to the four-bed room to join the others. Listened to a fine play on the wireless.

Sunday 19 October 1958

Pop, Mum, Uncle Dave and John came to see me. John brought two fine cigars. Shared them with Stubby in the evening – we had one each and stank the ward out.

Monday 20 October 1958

Wilkie came round and said he can do nothing more until the stitches are taken out. Domestic Ron Haylock wants me to knit a fancy cardigan for his little daughter. He gave me the pattern and I ordered the wool from OT. Looks a bit complicated but I'll do my best.

Tuesday 21 October 1958

After my blanket bath I started a new style basket – my own original design, weaving clockwise then anti-clockwise to create a zigzag pattern. OT asked me how I did it. Might patent it when I get out and make some serious bread.

Wednesday 22 October 1958

Clifford Glascoe visited me and stayed until 5:30 PM. Post arrived; a can of Anchor beer from Alan – wonderful. Had a laugh by kidding Orderly Dennis Wood he can sing – recorded his awful noise.

Thursday 23 October 1958

Waiting for the wool from OT so I can start work on the cardigan. Beat Stubby at chess. Another can of beer arrived, this time from John – I am blessed with such good friends and family.

Friday 24 October 1958

Beat Stubby again at chess. We pooled our winnings, bought a postal order and sent it to The Old Codgers at the Daily Mirror for their appeal. Still waiting for the wool and cane for baskets from OT. Ordered a general book on music from Foyle's in London. Be good to learn something while I'm here. Wrote to Alan at Hull who went to a pyjama dance at the university. Not impressed – I'm in pyjamas all the time, he can't beat that!

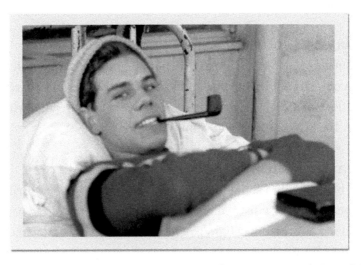

Here I am in the cold autumn air outside Denton Ward. Pipe full of 'baccy, bobble hat, warm sweater and a satisfied grin having just thrashed Stubby at chess – my chess set is in the little box on the covers.

Saturday 25 October 1958

Tried to chat up Nurse Christine Reynolds who just started on the ward as temporary staff. About time we had a bit of crumpet instead of the male Italian and English orderlies. I don't count Sister as crumpet; she can be a monster but fair enough, she has to control the ward.

Sunday 26 October 1958

Brian and Ron visited me. The ward Sister is back from holiday so we had better behave ourselves. Ray is sent home to Buntingford. The ward is a bit quieter now without his constant chatter.

Monday 27 October 1958

Wilkie came round and told the staff to take my weights off for one hour each day. Wish he'd take the bloody things off all the time. Had a bed bath but getting some very nasty bed sores on my back, being treated with a spirit rub. Mr Robinson with a very bad spine condition admitted.

Tuesday 28 October 1958

Finally got the wool from OT and started knitting the cardigan for domestic Ron's daughter with bunnies on it. Bit tricky but I can do it. Jimmy, a nice old chap, said he had 30 bob nicked from his bedside cabinet. I think he was mistaken – nobody here would do that.

Wednesday 29 October 1958

Mavis Peach – a patient of 15 in Astins Ward opposite – sent me a note to say hello written in Gaelic so I sent her one back in French. We can see each other across the divide between the two wards. She is in a full plaster boat from top to bottom and was in an iron lung at one time. Stubby Lagdon moved to a single room.

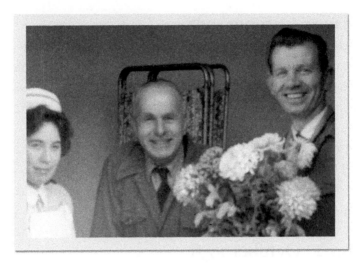

Domestics Rosemary, Tom Arnold and Ron Haylock.
I knitted a jumper for Ron's young daughter.

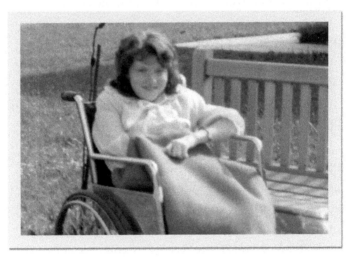

Mavis Peach from Astins Ward who spent
a lot of time in a plaster boat.

Thursday 30 October 1958

We all had a collection for Jimmy to restore his missing 30 shillings. He was very happy and thanked us all. A new bloke arrived in our room – Lionel Bryan, the first coloured bloke on the ward. Mavis keeps sending me letters; quote *"I'm crazy about Frankie Vaughan but am even more crazy about you"*. Bloody hell.

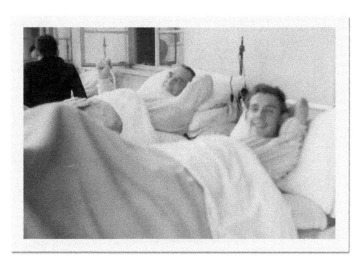

The bed patients were taken outside in all weathers as part of the treatment. Hughie is in the background chatting to one of them.

Friday 31 October 1958

Wrote to Mavis then continued knitting the cardigan – challenging but enjoyable. All of us on the ward started singing hymns and some Christmas Carols in the evening – not Christmas yet but it was just a bit of fun to relieve the boredom. Wrote to Alan at Hull thanking him for the booze and telling him about the letters Mavis keeps writing. I am glad if it makes her feel a bit happier.

Saturday 1 November 1958
Lionel Bryan gave me a fine cigar so I smoked it – very nice. I'm getting some more bad habits here.

Sunday 2 November 1958
Pop and Mum came to see me in the morning. Sister got mad because they stayed too long. The music book from Foyle's arrived free of charge – that was good of them.

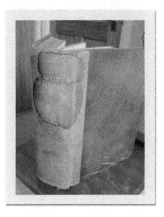

The music book that Foyle's sent me.
I still have it but it's a bit tatty now.

Monday 3 November 1958
Another letter arrived from Mavis. Finished the cardigan for Ron's young daughter. Listened to Brahms' *Cello Sonata op. 38* on the wireless.

Tuesday 4 November 1958
A bloke came to see me who was a former patient at the hospital with a similar complaint. He now works as a barber on the cruise ship Queen Elizabeth and seems fine. That was encouraging. Might apply for a job

on a cruise ship when I get out – teaching basket making and knitting perhaps. Sent a message to Ron that I had finished his daughter's cardigan. Was told he had an accident and was out cold for nearly four days. Will have to wait for him to recover. He had better – he owes me for the wool. A new bloke Michael Foster admitted to our room. Don't trust him; he's a bit creepy but maybe I will get used to him.

Wednesday 5 November 1958
Clifford Glascoe came to see me. In the evening, I asked Sister if we could go outside to see the fireworks as it is Guy Fawkes Night. She agreed but when we asked if we could stay out all night, she declined. Shame, it would be nice to lay out there in our beds all night spying on the nurses in Astins Ward. Maybe that's why Sister refused.

Thursday 6 November 1958
Made a start on another basket. Making a nice profit from them – I flog some of them to the hospital shop which seems to like my designs. Sold one to Clifford Glascoe. Should have given it to him really but I need the cash for more materials.

Friday 7 November 1958
A nurse ironed and wrapped the cardigan and I gave it to Ron for his daughter. It only cost me 10 shillings for the wool but he gave me a quid. Maybe I should take up knitting and baskets as a career. A can of Guinness arrived from Alan – most welcome.

Saturday 8 November 1958
Bought a poppy for Armistice Day. So far I have made and sold six baskets. I am enjoying doing this – creative and profitable. Weights taken off for two hours each day now.

Sunday 9 November 1958

Mickey Paris and Lulu visited me at 11:30 AM then they went to the pub and returned at 2:00 PM sneaking in a load of beer for me. Brian and Ann Cawthorne came later. She wanted to see my scar – not a pretty sight (the scar, not Ann).

Monday 10 November 1958

One of the orderlies told Sister that I seem unhappy on this ward. Don't know why, I am fine but would rather be home of course. Wilkie came round and saw me in the treatment room. He said I may be out by March.[1] Went back to the ward and got myself boozed up on the store of beer in my locker that Mickey brought in and Alan sent me from Hull. Drank three pints of Guinness, three bottles of light ale and half a bottle of rhubarb wine. Was sick all night – serves me right. Must have been the rhubarb wine. Wrote to Alan and sent him £5 until his grant comes through.

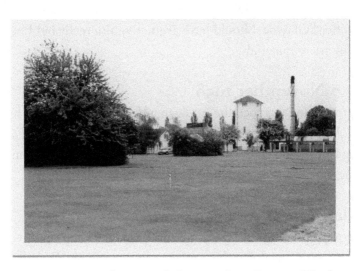

A view across the grounds but not from Denton Ward.

---

[1] Bit optimistic – I wasn't out until 19 May.

Tuesday 11 November 1958
Stubby Lagdon moved back to the room.

Wednesday 12 November 1958
Didn't get pushed outside today because it rained all day. Worked on three more small baskets.

Thursday 13 November 1958
Orderlies moved me, Bill, Stubby and Michael Foster into the next room. Can no longer see Mavis through the window from here. Maybe that's why they moved me.

Friday 14 November 1958
Made another herring-bone basket – still selling well.

Saturday 15 November 1958
Lost 5 bob on Hughie's roulette wheel – my profit on one basket. John visited at 7:00 PM – staying at Chelmsford.

Sunday 16 November 1958
Pop and Mum tried to get here in the morning but his beat-up old Austin car conked out. Brian came on his motorbike and brought with him the score of Brahms' cello sonata that I wanted.

Monday 17 November 1958
Wilkie came round and told the nurse to take off my weights for four hours every day. I organised a petition about the shortage of materials from OT and 16 patients signed it. I intend to give it to Mr Arthur Hadfield, the hospital secretary.

Tuesday 18 November 1958

Had another barney with the OT woman about the lack of materials for our baskets and things. Orderly Les Hackett lent me his music book to read.

Wednesday 19 November 1958

Harry Green returned to the ward with his arm in a sling. They had discharged him but he had problems. Pity he left because he gave me his ration of Guinness in exchange for me rolling his tobacco. Business is now resumed. Joe Trow has been called up for National Service and is in the RAF, hopefully not as a navigator – he tried to visit me today and only got as far as Chelmsford. He couldn't find Black Notley so gave up and went back.

Thursday 20 November 1958

New bloke Lionel Gosling arrived on the ward. The typed play *Black Notley Blues* arrived so we set the recording day for tomorrow afternoon. Started work on my 10th basket. Punch up between orderlies Ron Bowkett and Italian Joe.

Friday 21 November 1958

All the ten actors assembled in my room and I handed out the copied scripts of the play. Got quarter of the way through when I realised I had forgotten to turn on the tape recorder – so we had to start again! After we had finished, I spotted Mavis sitting in a wheelchair – she called across that she will write to me. Wrote to Alan thanking him for the postal order and the tin of Worthington.

Saturday 22 November 1958

Nurses Elaine and Betty from Astins Ward sneaked over at 8:30 PM and chatted to us. Just as well that Sister was off duty.

Sunday 23 November 1958

Pop and Mum visited at 11:30 AM and while they were here they listened to the play **Black Notley Blues** on the tape recorder. Mum said it's better than those on the tele such as *Emergency Ward 10* and *Doctor Kildare* and I should send it to the BBC. Well, mums always say things like that don't they?

Monday 24 November 1958

Nurse Margaret Cross from Astins sneaked over with a letter from Mavis at 6:20 AM asking for a photo of me. Wilkie came round and said weights can continue to come off for four hours each day. Bill Webb threw up over his bed – he has serious ulcer problems. Letter arrived from my penfriend Boyka in Yugoslavia.

Tuesday 25 November 1958

Played music on the tape recorder all day with earphones. Later on all the blokes assembled in my room and listened to our play – sounds pretty good. Everyone enjoyed it.

Wednesday 26 November 1958

Wrote to the Old Codgers in Live Letters (Daily Mirror) about our play. Thought they might be interested – but they weren't, the miserable old sods. Nothing yet from Mavis. Played rock'n'roll music on the tape recorder.

Thursday 27 November 1958

Very quiet today – still nothing from Mavis, maybe she is poorly. Started trying to compose a piano/cello sonata. Load of rubbish but it keeps me amused.

Friday 28 November 1958

Mr Duck, who owns a shop in the village and a taxi business, came round with the daily papers. I bought a box of chocolates from him and sent it over to Mavis with a get well soon note. Started making two hanging baskets for flowers – something different.

Saturday 29 November 1958

Letter at last from Mavis – as I thought, she has been quite ill. That's why she's here I guess.

Sunday 30 November 1958

Vera Fish and Brian turned up on his motorbike. They listened to our play. Chatted to Vera about her job.

Monday 1 December 1958

Wilkie did his rounds and my weights can come off for five hours daily now. Recorded Beethoven's *Eroica Symphony*.

Tuesday 2 December 1958

Mavis had her operation today. Bit of discomfort today – weights at a different angle, don't like it but have to put up with it. Made a small basket and started a bread roll basket for Clifford Glascoe.

Wednesday 3 December 1958

Stubby cheated at chess – threw a pillow at him. Clifford Glascoe didn't turn up today. Finished the bread roll basket. Listened to *Scheherazade* on the wireless.

Thursday 4 December 1958

Letter arrived from Joe Trow. Made two small baskets.

Friday 5 December 1958

Chess score: Stubby 17, me 5. Won 2/6d from Michael Foster because he broke the bet and shaved. He fancies a nurse in Astins Ward and wants to clean himself up a bit. Listened to Mozart's *Jupiter Symphony* on the wireless.

Saturday 6 December 1958

Started making a bunny for Orderly Jim Holt. Nurse Eunice Smith brought over a letter from Mavis. She is very unhappy about being restricted to a wheelchair – probably for life. Stubby threw me a grapefruit and it landed in my porridge spraying it everywhere. Had a fruit fight with Michael Foster across the ward. Got in big trouble with Sister – I didn't start it but got the blame anyway.

Sunday 7 December 1958

Pop, Mum and Ginger visited. Mum brought in some glass beads and strings so I could make some jewellery. Stubby's girl friend rushed in and put a screen around his bed. She told him his mum had just died. He was very upset so we left him alone. Won 8 bob at housy-housy.

Monday 8 December 1958

Saw Wilkie in the treatment room. Strep injections every other day from now. Weights off for 5 hours a day. Letters from Vera Fish and Mavis who is getting cross with me for chatting up the nurses. Wrote to Alan in Hull.

Tuesday 9 December 1958

Bill Webb's wife came in with home-made jam. I bought a jar to have with my toast. Had a bed bath but the sores are getting worse and painful. Letter from Maureen Copsey.

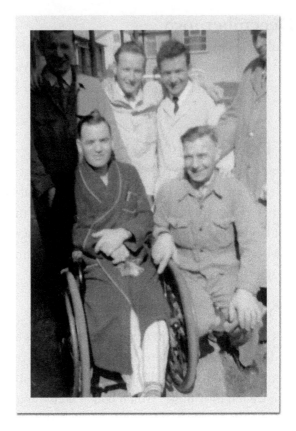

Back row left to right: Ron Haylock, Brian Hunnable,
Italian Tony but cannot remember the other one.
Front row: Bill Webb and Orderly Jim Holt.

Wednesday 10 December 1958

Sent off 7/6d to the Old Codgers Daily Mirror Christmas appeal.
Clifford Glascoe came in. Wrote Christmas cards.

Thursday 11 December 1958

Domestic Tom Arnold brought me a letter from Mavis. Made a small basket to put my cactus in. Wrote to Vera Fish. Had supper – soup tasted like boiled socks.

Friday 12 December 1958

A letter arrived for me and Stubby from the Daily Mirror addressed to the Chess Boys. Started work on a large basket. Heard that Mavis is going home tomorrow on respite leave, just for Christmas.

Saturday 13 December 1958

Mavis went before I could give her the letter so I posted it. John came to see me at 7:00 PM. He has a new bird – Angela.

Sunday 14 December 1958

Brian and Maureen Copsey visited me and brought a Giles cartoon book. Wrote to Valerie Keig at the HBS.

Monday 15 December 1958

Wilkie did his rounds – weights still off for only 5 hours a day. Had a pellet fight across the ward with Michael Foster and Stubby, and chucking wet newspapers at each other. Like a bunch of kids.

Tuesday 16 December 1958

Sister really had a go at us for making such a mess in the ward. She was furious and I don't blame her – we must behave ourselves in future. Started knitting a bobble hat for Vera Fish and making some jewellery from the stuff Mum brought in.

Wednesday 17 December 1958

Jock was discharged today. Cyril and Peter came in from another room on the ward as they were interested in buying some of my jewellery for Christmas presents – a new money-making racket. Haven't heard from Mavis yet.

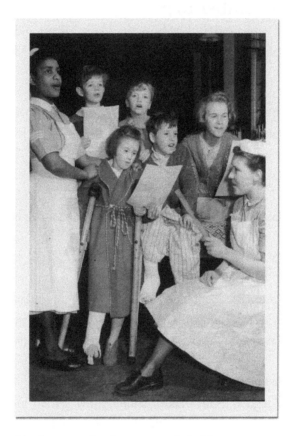

An old photograph of nurses and child patients singing
Christmas carols – bit before my time.

Thursday 18 December 1958

Made a waste paper basket on order. Nurses came over to talk about the candle club – lighting candles for Christmas. Letter from Gary Wooding.

Friday 19 December 1958

Still nothing from Mavis – wrote letters all afternoon and evening. We had a Christmas collection for Sister. I gave 2/6d – collected 3 quid in all.

Saturday 20 December 1958

Alan came to see me and while he was here some carol singers came round from the village.

Sunday 21 December 1958

Pop, Mum and Ginger came in at 11:45 AM and brought me Christmas presents and a nice cake. No visitors in the afternoon. Orderly Brian Hunnable bought some jewellery from me for gifts. Sent cards to all and £3 to Mum for the jewellery makings. I kept the profits. Played housy-housy and lost 6 bob. So much for profits.

Monday 22 December 1958

I've had 121 jabs so far – feel like a pin cushion. Wilkie came round and gave me marvellous news. The planks can be taken off the bed to make it softer to lay on – luxury, they've been on since 13 August making the bed hard like sleeping on concrete. Stockings, weights and strap can come off and I can get up after Christmas. May need another operation later. Christmas cards hung up all around my bed – and a letter from Boyka in Yugoslavia. Happy days are here again!

Tuesday 23 December 1958

Christmas card arrived from Mavis. I have 30 cards now hanging around my bed. We all had our beds pushed outside and we sang carols to the nurses as they passed by the ward.

Wednesday 24 December 1958

Big fuss because Deputy Matron Miss Palmer was due to visit the wards in the afternoon. During the evening a load of nurses arrived holding candles and singing Christmas carols – I recorded them on my Grundig. Clifford Glascoe popped in – good to see him. Nurse Eunice Smith and her friend came in and had a drink with us. Orderlies Les Hackett and Jim Brown pushed Michael's and Stubby's beds across the ward and we all had a booze up until 3:00 in the morning.

Thursday 25 December 1958

Christmas Day – merry Christmas to one and all! Nurse Eunice Smith returned after breakfast and clutching a bunch of mistletoe, went round the ward snogging the patients. Staff Nurse Taffy Price had a hangover so he went to sleep in a spare bed in one of the rooms. Dr Brahma came round the ward but he was a bit sloshed so he legged it as soon as Wilkie arrived. Deputy Matron came back and asked to hear the recording of the nurses singing carols on my recorder. She asked if I can transfer it to vinyl records for the hospital. I will find out. Evening, Nurse Christine Reynolds bounced onto the ward sloshed and sprawled herself across my bed until she was much later chucked out by the night nurse – pity. She turned up again to apologise for her behaviour. I assured her it wasn't necessary and she is welcome to come back any time. Michael Foster in the bed opposite spent the evening snogging Nurse Frances. Well, it is Christmas – the season of goodwill to all patients and their nurses.

Friday 26 December 1958

The nurses came round again but Sister wouldn't let them in. Mickey Paris and Lulu visited me in the afternoon – John and Alan arrived later. Great to see them all on Boxing Day. The doctors came to hear the carols on the tape recorder. Evening, Nurse Brenda Lomax came to see Michael Foster. She put a screen around his bed and stayed most of the night. She went early morning before the day staff came on. I can guess what they were up to.

Saturday 27 December 1958

Catering manager Mr Pirie came in with his wife to listen to the carols on the recorder – everyone wants to hear them. Nurse Brenda Lomax crept over from Astins Ward to see Michael Foster again. While they were behind the screen, I joined Bill and Stubby in a Guinness booze up – had four pints each saved up from our daily rations.

Sunday 28 December 1958

Ron and Brian visited in the morning – no visitors in the afternoon. Len and Hughie back from respite leave. Busted my glasses and stuck the bits together with sticky tape.

Monday 29 December 1958

Mavis's 16th birthday. Sent a parcel of goodies to her home in Staffordshire. Wilkie came round and said I could get up for two hours each day in a wheelchair. Got out of bed but felt dizzy so went back in – it felt strange after spending over four and a half months lying in bed. Nurse Eunice Smith crept over from Astins Ward and told me that Nurse Christine Reynolds has written to me.

Tuesday 30 December 1958

Finally got out of bed from 2:00 pm until 5:30 pm. Felt nervous
but excited at being vertical at last. Drove around the wards in my
wheelchair and met patients I had never seen before in the other rooms.
Weight gone down to 8 stone 8 lbs. Went to the day room and played
dominoes with Stubby. Letters from Vera Fish, Nurse Christine Reynolds
and from Mavis.

Wednesday 31 December 1958

Got up for another two hours and played cards with Stubby and
Michael. Len West was discharged and went home – had a booze up
with him before he left. Listened to Schubert's *Trout Quintet* on the
wireless. Orderly Les Hackett brought in some home-made wine which
he shared out to celebrate New Year's Eve. Nurse Jean popped in to see
us and had a glass.

Thursday 1 January 1959

The hospital van picked up me and Stubby and took us to the social
centre cinema to see *Cockleshell Heroes*. Fine nurses in there. Feel a
bit stronger and confident about getting around now. Started knitting
a jumper for Mum.

Friday 2 January 1959

Knitted all morning then went in a wheelchair to the social centre for
the staff concert. Doctors, nurses and some patients put on a show for us.
The choir sang some songs including *Cherry Ripe* – sounded more like
Cherry Tripe but we all enjoyed it. Returned to the ward in the back of a
truck. Evening, played chess with Stubby.

Saturday 3 January 1959

Watched the tele in the day room with Bill then went to see Eddie Fredericks – I felt bad and nearly passed out so went back to bed. Got up again later and went round the rooms chatting. Snowing like mad outside. Mavis back from respite today.

Sunday 4 January 1959

Pop, Mum and Ginger came in at 11:45 AM. Brought me some warm clothes so I could go out in the cold. Did more knitting in the afternoon. Nurse Eunice popped over to see me and said Mavis has heard about what I got up to with Christine Reynolds over Christmas and she is not pleased at all. Thought I'd better lie low for a while so got up and went round the ward chatting.

Monday 5 January 1959

Wilkie came round – still up for only two hours each day, no more. Orderly Dennis Wood pushed me in a wheelchair to see the optician to get new glasses. Dennis had to leave me there so I tried to get back to the ward myself in the wheelchair. I got stuck in the snow and had to wait in the freezing cold for someone to come by and help. Eventually a new nurse Ruthie Wilson found me and pushed me back. She said when I get up properly I should come and visit her in the nurses' home. I rather fancy Ruthie with her auburn hair. Must try and find where the nurses' home is. When I got back there was a parcel on my bed – an inscribed cigarette case from Mavis. No good to me as I only smoke a pipe but a kind thought anyway. Tried to send her a message to thank her but the nurse said she's asleep waiting for an operation tomorrow.

Tuesday 6 January 1959

Mavis went for her operation at 11:00 AM returning at 3:00 PM. She was once in an iron lung so I am concerned. In the afternoon I went round the grounds in my wheelchair. Later in the evening I asked Sister if I could pop across to see Mavis. She said she will ask Matron. Why ask Matron when I could just sneak across? Stubby gave me a Jerry Lewis haircut because I was out when the barber called.

Wednesday 7 January 1959

Sent Boyka one of my made-up necklaces. Wilkie came round with a Japanese surgeon and told Stubby he could now get up for two hours in a chair. He is shorter than I thought – maybe that's why they call him Stubby, unless there is another reason! Alan visited in the afternoon and took me for a ride round the grounds in the wheelchair. I asked him to phone Clifford Glascoe not to come today. Evening, played draughts with Stubby.

Thursday 8 January 1959

Pop sold his Austin and bought a 1948 Hillman Minx. Went to the social centre with Stubby in wheelchairs to see *Seven Waves Away*. Nurse Julie from Astins Ward pushed me back to the ward. Don't know how Stubby got back. Evening, wandered round the rooms then when things were quiet, I tried to go outside to see Mavis on Astins Ward. Couldn't get in but Nurse Julie said Mavis has got my photo by her bed – if it makes her happy that's fine.

Friday 9 January 1959

Knitted all morning and got up in the afternoon. Wandered round the rooms with Stubby chatting to other patients. Saw Mavis out of the window and gave her a wave. Played pontoon with Hughie Keating. Evening, listened to Prokofiev's *Classical Symphony* and Beethoven's *Eroica*.

When it was quiet, Nurse Julie knocked on the window and beckoned me over to Astins Ward. She had put a screen around Mavis's bed and said I could stay for a while, but must not tell anyone or we will all be in big trouble. Mavis was covered in plaster lying in bed but she was very happy to see me and chat for a while. I gave her a little kiss then crept back to Denton Ward. Vera Fish wrote to say that her sister Margaret had bought my Soprani accordion for £4.

Saturday 10 January 1959

Went out in the snow with Stubby to a concert in the social centre. It was another cabaret show starring the staff and patients. Evening, watched Marty Wilde and Cliff Richard in *Oh Boy!* on the tele with Bill and Michael, then resumed my knitting.

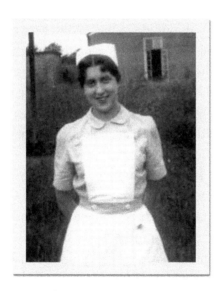

*I cannot be certain but this is possibly
Nurse Julie from Astins Ward, one of the nurses
who encouraged me to sneak over to see Mavis.*

Sunday 11 January 1959

Got up early and delivered Michael's letter to Irish Nurse Janet Warner who he is trying to get off with. Brian came in at 12 o'clock. After he went, I got up and went out on my own. Mavis has moved to another room so I bunked out to see her in my wheelchair.

Monday 12 January 1959

Sister found out about me visiting Mavis and reminded me it is forbidden to fraternise with nurses or patients of the opposite sex. The optician arrived and measured me up for new glasses. Wilkie came round and said I could try and use crutches for four hours each day. A bloke from physiotherapy brought a pair round for me. I tried to stand very carefully but it was tricky – so different being vertical rather than horizontal.

Tuesday 13 January 1959

They pushed all the beds outside in the cold so I stayed under the covers and knitted. Still a bit nervous about using the crutches so I went round the grounds in a wheelchair with Stubby. Saw Nurse Eunice outside Astins Ward – I asked her how was Mavis. She is doing OK but still cannot use her hands properly, that is why Mavis dictates letters to Eunice for me. Went back to the ward and made an apple pie bed for Hughie.

Wednesday 14 January 1959

Stubby's 26th birthday today. Did some knitting then Clifford Glascoe came in. He's a nice chap and spent some time telling me how the stock market worked – bull and bear markets etc. Wilkie came round and told Stubby he can go home tomorrow. Losing my chess partner, but a new bloke arrived – Derek King a solicitor. He seemed a bit lost so we played chess together.

Thursday 15 January 1959

Went over to OT to buy some wool. Stubby's dad arrived to collect him in a car at 2:00 PM. We all said goodbye to him. I went to a concert in the afternoon in my wheelchair. Michael Foster was pushed there on a stretcher as he is still in a plaster boat. An old chap David Taylor moved into Stubby's vacated bed. Nurse Eunice crept in after lights out to see Michael. I went to sleep before she left – she was gone before the day staff arrived.

Friday 16 January 1959

Another patient died today – Mr Elam. Finished knitting Mum's sweater then explored the grounds again in my wheelchair. Letter from Maureen Cooper from HBS. I miss Stubby but I'm sure I will find someone else to torment.

Saturday 17 January 1959

Got up – Bill in the day room watching tele. Now I've finished Mum's sweater I decided to try something difficult and knit Mavis a pair of gloves. Shouted across to Mavis and told her I will knit her a present.

Sunday 18 January 1959

No visitors today – too cold. After lights out I sneaked over to Astins Ward in my wheelchair through the snow to see Mavis. On the way back the wheelchair got stuck in the snow and one of the nurses had to come and dig me out. Sister found out about it and had another go at me. This is becoming a habit.

Monday 19 January 1959

Mr Duck is late with the newspapers. Dr Raymond, a psychiatrist, admitted as a patient today. Wilkie saw me in the day room – he wants to operate on me again. I think he said a displacement osteotomy. Orderly Dennis Wood helped me get into a real bath – so nice to have a proper bath instead of those bed baths. Went to OT and found an old piano there so I had a go at playing it. Still remember some classical pieces by Beethoven, Chopin, Schubert and Liszt. The OT staff were astonished that I could play so well after having been in bed for so long. Evening, listened to Puccini's *Madame Butterfly* on the wireless earphones.

Tuesday 20 January 1959

Bought some wool and a pattern from OT to make gloves for Mavis and a Mickey Mouse cuddly toy. Patient Ted Hoskins showed me a letter from Nurse Christine Reynolds.

Wednesday 21 January 1959

Parcel of goodies arrived from Mum. Palled up with Irish Michael Flaherty from another room. He was allowed up for the first time today. Went out in our wheelchairs first to the social centre then we found the nurses' home. We couldn't get the wheelchairs up the steps so we chatted outside to student nurses Carol and Linda. Then Sister Bartholomew suddenly appeared and asked what were we doing at the nurses' home. I said *"Nurses' home? I thought this was the Black Notley Museum"*. She got angry and threatened to sling us out. A porter pushed Michael back to the ward – I had to get back myself.

Thursday 22 January 1959

Heard on the news that racing driver Mike Hawthorn had been killed. Continued making the Mickey Mouse toy then went to the social centre with Irish Michael to see *Red Beret* starring Alan Ladd. Chatted up nurses from Ward 3 but had to watch out for Sister. Got in trouble with Staff Nurse Taffy Price for being out of the ward after 8:00 PM.

Friday 23 January 1959

Went with Irish Michael to the phone box, which is out of bounds, as he wanted to phone someone in Ireland. Showed him how to tap out the number to get a free call – he was amazed. I returned to the ward as fast as I could to cover for him. Evening, took the finished Mickey Mouse to Astins Ward and left it with the duty nurse to give to Mavis. Crept back to the ward but Taffy Price caught me and said I must not leave the ward after 8 o'clock. He wrote something about it in the report book.

Saturday 24 January 1959

Sister found out about me leaving the ward after 8:00 PM so I am in trouble with her again. Nurse Margaret Lever from Astins called me to say when things are quiet she will flash a torch and I can creep over there to see Mavis. At 9:00 PM when things had settled down, Nurse Margaret flashed the torch so I left my bed and crept over to Astins for half an hour, but the night nurse Jim Brown saw me and noted in the report book that I was out until 9:30 PM. Later on Nurse Margaret flashed the torch again so I crept over there and didn't get back until midnight. This time Jim Brown didn't see me so the report still said I was back at 9:30 PM, which was bad enough anyway.

Sunday 25 January 1959

When Sister saw the report book, she came round to my bed in a foul
mood and really lashed into me, and said I was confined to the ward
until further notice. She also told Pop and Mum when they visited me
in the afternoon. They thought it was rather funny but daren't say so
to Sister. I had to send a note to Mavis to tell her I am grounded for a
while – confined to barracks, in disgrace.

Monday 26 January 1959

New glasses arrived – paid optician 6/2d for them. Wilkie came round
in the afternoon and said my second operation will be next week or
the week after. I asked Sister if I could go to OT to buy some wool.
She agreed as long as I went with someone and came straight back.
So I went with Irish Michael who went to the forbidden phone box
to 'tap out' Ireland. When we got back to the ward I told Sister that
Michael had been with me all the time.

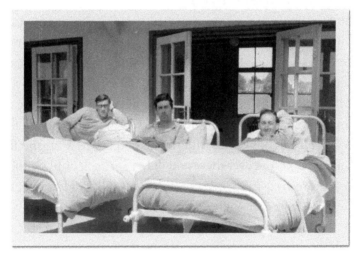

Derek King (solicitor), Alan Jones (fantasist) and Jerry Smith.

Tuesday 27 January 1959

Got dressed and went to the social centre with Irish Michael having cleared it with Sister. Chatted up the nurses from Ward 2. Had to keep a watch out for Sister – don't want to get caught fraternising again. I behaved myself in the evening, listening to Beethoven's *Piano Concerto no. 4* on the wireless.

Wednesday 28 January 1959

Received a letter from Margaret Rose Faulkner from Ireland – just another penfriend. Stayed in bed all afternoon expecting Clifford Glascoe but he was unable to come. A new buxom blonde woman called Freda arrived on the ward with a German woman, both employed as cleaners. I saw Bill chatting up Freda who seems very street-wise but a bit simple. I went in the kitchen and helped the German girl with the washing up. Sent some comics over to Mavis to cheer her up as my nocturnal visits are over – well, for the time being.

Thursday 29 January 1959

Got up in the afternoon to visit OT but had a headache so went back to bed. Made a waste basket from cane. Irish Michael went to the social centre for a game of billiards.

Friday 30 January 1959

Went to the social centre on my own – it's OK with Sister now – as long as I behave myself. After supper I listened to Berlioz on the wireless. Intended to bunk out to see Mavis but Nurse Margaret wasn't on duty with her torch.

Saturday 31 January 1959

My hands are getting sore from leaning on those crutches so I spoke to Dr Brahma about it. I'm finding it difficult to open my bottles of Guinness and that's serious. Went round the grounds on my own and sat on a bench outside Ward 8, the first ward I was admitted to. Back on Denton Ward I went to bed but woke up at 9:30 PM with a bright light flashing in my eyes. It was Nurse Margaret with her torch again. So I crept out of bed and went over to see Mavis and didn't get back until midnight. No sign of Jim Brown this time – I had got away with it.[2]

Sunday 1 February 1959

After breakfast I got up and hopped over to the social centre. Afternoon, Brian and Vera Fish came to see me on his motorbike.

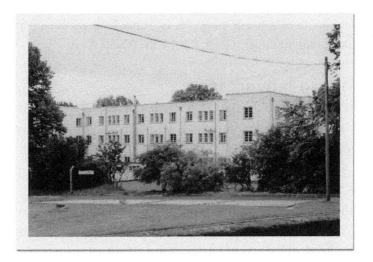

Here is the nurses' home – strictly out of bounds of course.

---

[2] …or so I thought at the time.

Monday 2 February 1959

Saw Wilkie in the day room who told me the next operation will be on Thursday. Crutches now replaced with sticks. Can now use the flush bog instead of bed pans for a few days. Saw Julie Birch (friend of Mavis) outside who said Mavis is not well and has the screens around her all the time.

Tuesday 3 February 1959

Orderly Roy Gatwood helped to scrub me down and prepare me for the op. Wrote letters in the afternoon. Back on strep tomorrow. The barber came round the wards.

Wednesday 4 February 1959

Clifford Glascoe phoned. Orderlies Dennis Wood and Brian Hunnable bathed me again – never been so clean. I have every confidence in Wilkie and his medical staff but I always feel a bit nervous before an operation.

Thursday 5 February 1959

My ear is buzzing like crazy but I didn't say anything about it as the pre-med may have triggered the tinnitus as it did last time. Staff Nurse George Moase moved me into a single room and smothered me with iodine, then pushed me across the grounds to the theatre at 2:00 PM. As I passed the wards, I saw some of the nurses waving to me. Hope they weren't waving goodbye! Next thing I vaguely remember was being pushed across the grounds back to the ward then being lifted off the trolley into a bed in a single room. I am now in plaster from my tits to my toes.

Friday 6 February 1959

Felt worse than the previous operation. Nasty pain and constant headache. Wilkie came to see me with Dr Brahma several times. Clothes taken away so I couldn't get up, not that I felt like it. Then worse still, Jim Brown the male nurse, came in after lights out and tried it on while I was still semi-conscious, so I rang the alarm bell. He backed off and said if I tell anyone, he will tell Sister I had been out until midnight last Saturday. So the ratbag must have seen me creep back to the ward after visiting Mavis last time. He escaped through the French windows before the duty night nurse arrived responding to my alarm call. I was tempted to tell her about Jim but decided to keep quiet as I now have one over on him. Horrible man – ugh!

Saturday 7 February 1959

Still felt lousy and haven't eaten anything since before the operation. Received a card and letter from Mavis. Evening, some of the other patients popped in to see me.

Sunday 8 February 1959

Pop, Mum and Ginger visited me at 11:30 PM. I asked Mum to go over to see Mavis and give her the gloves I had knitted. Pop went round to see Bill Webb who had no visitors. After they went, Mickey Paris and Gary Wooding arrived on a scooter. Still feel rough but getting better.

Monday 9 February 1959

Got a bloody great bed sore on my bum – Staff Nurse George Moase lifted me up and shoved an air ring under me to relieve the pain of it. Apart from that I feel better.

Tuesday 10 February 1959

Sister and Taffy Price came in and cleaned me up in the morning. Obviously Jim Brown – worried that I might grass him up – had not reported to Sister that I was off the ward until midnight or she would have clobbered me by now. They pushed me back to my room with the other three. Tried a glass of Guinness but it didn't stay down very long.

Wednesday 11 February 1959

Was awake most of last night with a headache. Finally got to sleep around 4:30 AM. Clifford Glascoe came to see me in the afternoon and we had an interesting talk about mechanised branches. Bed sore really playing up – it is treated four times a day with a spirit rub.

Thursday 12 February 1959

Nothing very exciting today – my wings have been clipped again and I am back in bed covered in plaster. It itches like buggery under the plaster so I shoved a knitting needle down there to try and relieve the itch but I made it worse by breaking the skin.

Friday 13 February 1959

Received a Valentine card from Irish Margaret in Dublin. OT gave me some material to make a teddy bear.

Saturday 14 February 1959

Michael Foster got some help to get him in a wheelchair and sneak over to Astins to see Nurse Margaret. Valentine card arrived from Vera. Bum still sore – rubbed with spirit three times a day. Dr Brahma left the hospital today.

Sunday 15 February 1959

Brian, Ron and Maureen Copsey came to see me. Brian and Ron
went to the social centre – left alone with Maureen. Looked out of
the window and saw Mavis scowling at me. Too bad, she should have
sent me a Valentine card.

Monday 16 February 1959

Wilkie said the plaster will be changed in 10 days' time. A letter
arrived from Mavis asking *"Who was that blonde bird by your bed?"*
What's she worried about – Maureen was by the bed, not in it? A new
doctor, Dr De Rozka came round the ward. He is Persian – we call
him 'Persian Pete'.

Tuesday 17 February 1959

Worked all morning on the teddy bear – called it Weena from HG Wells'
Time Machine book. My sore bum is a bit better now after all the
treatment, but is still being rubbed three or four times a day. Jim Brown
is back on day duty but keeps well away from me fortunately. I should
now be able to get away with bunking out while he is on duty!

Wednesday 18 February 1959

Finished off Weena but lost the sewing needle in my bed somewhere.
Called the orderly who said it's dangerous losing a needle in the bed so
he lifted me out and searched for it. Couldn't find it anywhere – maybe
it fell on the floor or down the gap between me and the plaster. Just have
to be careful and wait and see if it turns up.

Thursday 19 February 1959

Irish Margaret from Dublin sent me a parcel of magazines to read –
very good of her. Message from Astins that Mavis is fed up as I haven't
been over there for a while. Can't help it, I'm stuck in this sodding bed.

I still cannot find that needle anywhere – I wonder if it's in Weena's stuffing, now there's a thought. Michael bunked over to see Nurse Margaret again. That ratbag always gets away with it.

Friday 20 February 1959
Wilkie came round with three student doctors and examined me. In the next bed Bill's ulcer burst and he was carted off for urgent treatment.

Saturday 21 February 1959
Other patients were pushed outside but I stayed behind to listen to *Paul Temple* on the wireless. Started knitting some more gloves – maybe for Vera this time. Mavis sent a note then went home at 12 o'clock for a month's respite. Feel rotten about neglecting her but I can't help it – I'm stuck in bed. Listened to *The Annoying Dr. Clutterhouse* on the wireless.

Sunday 22 February 1959
Pop, Mum, Ginger and Uncle Les visited me at 11:30 AM. Nice to see them all. Wrote some letters in the afternoon and listened to my tape recorder. Michael Foster borrowed it to play to Nurse Margaret. I thought he had better things to do with her.

Monday 23 February 1959
Went down for an x-ray. I took Weena with me and asked the radiologist if she would x-ray the teddy bear in case the missing needle is inside the stuffing. She was in good humour and said she had never x-rayed a teddy bear before. She laid it down on the table and told it to hold its breath and not move – all good fun. When the x-ray plate was developed it showed the needle in the stuffing, but I stopped short of sending it to the operating theatre to have it surgically removed, preferring instead to use a crochet needle. Bill Webb is now out of his plaster boat and hopes to go home shortly. Finished knitting one of the gloves – tricky stuff.

Tuesday 24 February 1959

Tom Beard is back from his operation. Michael moved over the other side of the room with Bill in his place and Tom next to me. Hughie Keating and Paddy Kelly are now back on the ward after respite.

Wednesday 25 February 1959

Freda the cleaner came round and announced that she is in the family way by a bloke in the village. Afternoon, John visited me and brought some eggs. He phoned Clifford Glascoe to say not to come in today. Michael had a row with Geoff Purl, Ray Clark and Peter. Don't know what all that was about. Dave Taylor's operation tomorrow.

Thursday 26 February 1959

Went down to the plaster room to have it removed and replaced with a shorter one. Was told I can get up tomorrow – great. A new doctor came to see us in the evening. He listened to our play on the tape recorder.

Friday 27 February 1959

Was pushed outside but the new plaster is bloody uncomfortable. Michael Foster went home for a while on respite – that's a relief, he's a real pain in the bum, worse than my bed sores. Tom Beard moved over the other side. Afternoon, got up for two hours in a chair. Nice to get up again even though it is uncomfortable with the plaster but I am sure to get used to it.

Saturday 28 February 1959

Wrote some letters then got up at 3:30 PM and went to chat with Geoff Purl. Went back to bed at 5:30 PM – that's my ration for the day.

Sunday 1 March 1959

Got up at 11:30 AM and wandered round the ward chatting to Alan Jones. He has a thing about black knickers with red cherries on them – funny bloke. Afternoon, Brian and Vera arrived by motorbike. Vera looks cute wearing a crash helmet. After they went, I played with the Grundig and recorded some of the patients chatting.

Monday 2 March 1959

Wilkie came round and told me to carry on, whatever that means. Afternoon, Orderly Mrs Harris gave me a bed bath. If she wasn't so butch I might fancy her.

Tuesday 3 March 1959

Knitted all day but got up for two hours in the afternoon. The dressing gown that Pop lent me has disappeared. He brought it back from the war and wants it returned.

Wednesday 4 March 1959

Messed around outside in the morning. Me, Geoff, Paul and Peter sang rock'n'roll songs across to Astins Ward to entertain the nurses and patients there. Clifford Glascoe came to see me in the afternoon. He is very friendly and worldly-wise, and teaches me a lot in his intelligent conversation. Teddy Hoskins is back on the ward.

Thursday 5 March 1959

Got up and stayed up all day messing around on the ward and chatting to the patients. Not much else doing.

Friday 6 March 1959

Doreen Price phoned. Got up at 7:00 AM and did some maths problems with Bert and Charlie Squires. Had to do some knee bending exercises – getting more mobile.

Saturday 7 March 1959

Wilkie came round and told me to get up a bit more. Went down to the day room to see what's on the tele – watched *Cheyenne* then the tele broke down.

Sunday 8 March 1959

Mothering Sunday today. Pop, Mum and Ginger came to see me in the morning. Pop reminded Sister about the missing dressing gown. She will make enquiries about it. Had a kip in the afternoon then got up at 6:30 PM and wandered round the ward. Bit frustrated that I cannot leave the ward yet.

Monday 9 March 1959

Wilkie came round while we were in our beds outside. He told me to get up for only two hours each day in a chair and crutches. Bit like old times. Got up for a while and helped some old boy get a pan from bed pan alley.

Tuesday 10 March 1959

Received a letter with photo from Boyka in Yugoslavia – she is a gorgeous bird. Alan Jones grabbed Weena the teddy bear and threw her over to Astins Ward where a little girl patient wearing a red dress picked it up. I was really pissed off with Alan but relented when I saw the girl's parents smiling and waving their thanks. I wrote a letter for Tom Beard to his firm because Tom couldn't write very well. Wrote to Alan in Hull who had just given blood – wonder if I will get it.

Wednesday 11 March 1959

Sister came round and told me off because my brother Brian had written to Arthur Hadfield (hospital secretary) about the missing dressing gown. I knew nothing about him writing. So Mr Hadfield came in to see me – such a lot of fuss. Afternoon, went over to Astins with Domestic Rosemary and got orders for some baskets from Mrs Cook. Asked Ron Haylock to get me a frame for Boyka's photo.

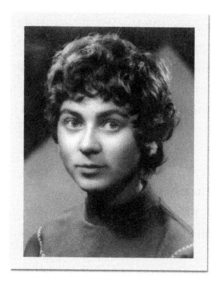

This is my penfriend Boyka Ceremov from Novi Sad in Yugoslavia.
We wrote to each other for a long time and exchanged presents.
I displayed this photo by my bed and told everyone she is my
girlfriend. They must have wondered why she never visited me.
She studied to become a doctor – wish she would get a job here
in Black Notley. I wouldn't want to go home!

Thursday 12 March 1959

Got up at 1:30 PM and went over to the social centre in a wheelchair with Lionel Gosling and Peter Collinson, the new bloke. Peter is a man of the world and I am hugely impressed when he said he had been to America. Never met anyone before who had visited America. We hung around the social centre chatting to the nurses as they went past. When I got back to the ward, Sister had another nag at me about Brian's letter to Mr Hadfield.

Friday 13 March 1959

Got up at 2:00 PM and it was sunny so I went down to the social centre and sat on the wall outside with Peter Collinson and Geoff Purl watching the nurses go by. Sister was still grumpy with me over that dressing gown. Evening, showed the other patients some conjuring tricks I had remembered. They pretended to be impressed. Recorded Peter and Geoff singing in the day room. Had a good laugh. Ron brought in a frame for Boyka's photo. I put it in and displayed it on my bedside cabinet.

Saturday 14 March 1959

Wilkie did his rounds then I did mine, around the grounds all afternoon in a wheelchair. Chatted to the nurses and patients in Ward 2. Evening, recorded the boys singing in the day room. Michael Foster is back again and he wasted no time in getting Nurse Margaret to come over and see him.

Sunday 15 March 1959

Had a pillow fight with Orderly Brian Hunnable. Later on Pop and Ginger visited me – no Vera this time. Evening, did some more recordings of the boys singing and telling jokes.

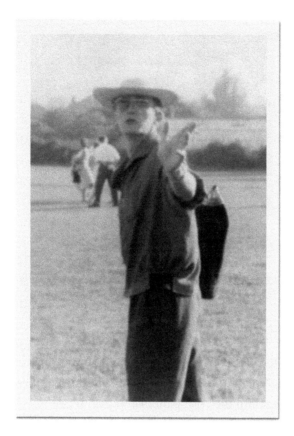

Peter Collinson who had been to America. He got up
to no good with Nurse Carol in Snakey Lane near
the hospital. That's what he told me anyway.

Monday 16 March 1959

Quiet morning except the Italian orderlies taught me a few swear words
in Italian – maybe useful one day. Evening, went to see the Irish bloke
Edward Leech just admitted. Wilkie came round but he only saw the
new patients.

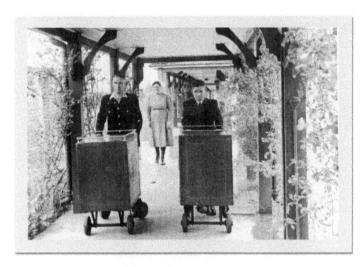

The Covered Walkway with porters delivering the meals to the wards.
Photo: © Nursing Times.

Tuesday 17 March 1959

Wrote a few letters then got up and wandered around wearing my new knitted scarf. Celebrated St Patrick's Day by lighting candles and having a few Guinnesses with the Irish patients.

Wednesday 18 March 1959

Staff Nurse George Moase trimmed my plaster and found a new bed sore – very painful. One of the patients ran a book for horse racing so I had a gamble and bet a shilling on Marshal Pil and it won. Then the mother of the girl wearing the red dress who had Weena came to thank me in the day room and gave me an ounce of St Bruno pipe tobacco. Recorded the boys singing again but they wanted an instrument so I wrote home to bring in my banjo. Mum said she couldn't find it which is a pity. I bet Sister was behind that: *"No banjos on the ward please!"*

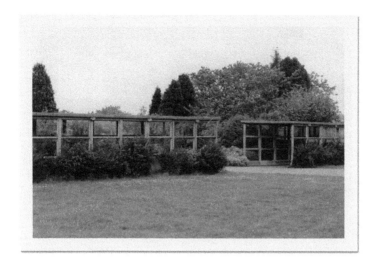

The Covered Walkway again: I took both these photos during my visit in 1997 just before the hospital closed down.

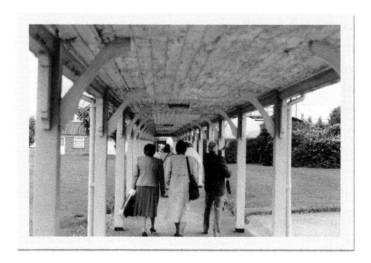

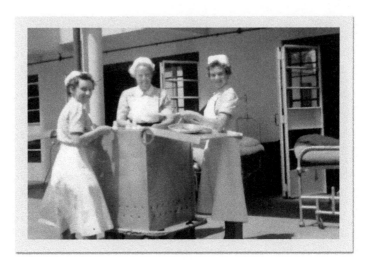

The nurses serving grub to the patients.
Photo: Courtesy of Marjorie Smith (née Tiley),
former patient and fellow student at Tottenham County School.

Thursday 19 March 1959

Went to the social centre cinema to see the film *Interpol*. I went in a wheelchair while Michael Foster and Bill Webb were pushed there in stretchers by orderlies. I then went to OT to ask them to iron my new scarf. Saw a new nurse in Astins – will find out more.

Friday 20 March 1959

Went to a concert in the social centre with Bill on a stretcher. Fine show, again starring some staff and patients. Went back and recorded Holst's *Planets*.

Saturday 21 March 1959

Put 10 bob on a horse in the Grand National but lost – my luck has run out. Afternoon, quite sunny so went out on my own to the nurses' home and saw Ruthie Wilson – a fine Irish nurse. We chatted for an hour. I remembered her from January when she pushed me back to the ward through the snow. She invited me in and introduced me to other nurses who made some tea. Went back to the ward but didn't tell anyone about where I had been, especially that rat Michael Foster – I'll keep that one to myself.

Sunday 22 March 1959

Pop, Mum, Ginger and Uncle Fred came to see me. After they had gone I went out again in the wheelchair to find Ruthie Wilson. Couldn't see her anywhere so went back to the ward. Later on I went out again and ran into Nurse Christine Reynolds, the one who landed on my bed at Christmas. She pushed my chair over to the benches near the tennis courts where we got better acquainted.

Monday 23 March 1959

Went out in a wheelchair towards the nurses' home. Patient Ted Hoskins saw me and we decided to risk it and leave the hospital grounds – strictly forbidden of course. He pushed me past the nurses' home and through the main gates towards the village shops. We saw Lionel Bryan on the way; he had also bunked out. Also saw Nurses Christine Reynolds and Wendy walking together towards the gate. I asked them to keep quiet about seeing us. Back on the ward I wrote to Ruthie Wilson suggesting we meet up on the bench by the tennis courts.

Tuesday 24 March 1959

Wilkie came round and said the foot rotation plaster could be removed and I can get up on crutches for half a day now. Michael Foster is also allowed up so watch out Nurse Margaret. Afternoon, went out on crutches with Michael in his wheelchair to the Memorial Hall. Didn't take him anywhere near the nurses' home! Evening, Alan visited me and I saw him in the day room – he will come again tomorrow so is probably staying at Aunt Lill's. Letter arrived from Ruthie Wilson.

Wednesday 25 March 1959

Alan returned and he pushed me to the social centre where we sat on the wall chatting up some nurses. Saw Nurse Ruthie Wilson and arranged to meet her tomorrow. Evening, Michael Foster on his crutches tried to get off with Freda but it didn't work out because Mrs Harris was on duty. Wilkie should have castrated him.

Thursday 26 March 1959

Went to the plaster room for a replacement then stayed in bed. Can get up tomorrow and try to get around. Ruthie Wilson wrote and said her shift has changed. Played my tape recorder in the evening. Bill Webb got up at last.

Friday 27 March 1959

Got up and carefully tried to walk a bit – went to the gym and they measured me, 5'11". Went to the phone box to 'tap out' Clifford Glascoe. Saw nurses Christine, Ruthie and Wendy on the way back – chatted them up. Irish Michael caught up with me and we went off with Christine Reynolds. Evening, played chess with Charlie Squires.

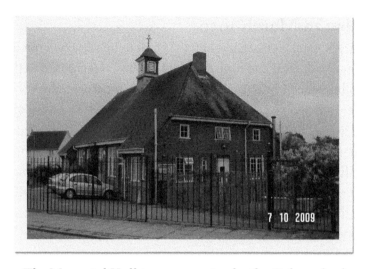

The Memorial Hall is now a centre for the Colourwheel Montessori Nursery.

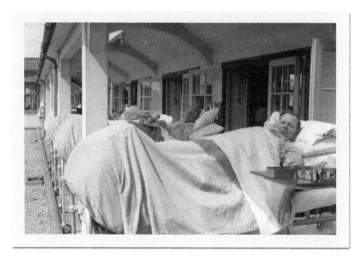

Charlie Squires outside Denton Ward. His chess set is on the table beside the bed.

Saturday 28 March 1959

Morning, got up at 9:00 AM and hopped around the ward on crutches. Afternoon, got dressed and bunked out of the hospital grounds to the village to buy some Easter eggs. Asked the duty nurse on Astins if I could go on the ward and give an egg to Ruthie. She said OK so I went on the ward, found Ruthie and gave her an egg and she gave me a letter arranging to see me tomorrow. Back on the ward, I watched tele until 8:30 PM. Jim Brown came on duty – we think he had been drinking. I bunked out at 10:30 PM to see Nurse Margaret in Astins – that will upset Mr Foster! I stayed with her until 1:00 AM then crept back across the grass to bed. Jim Brown saw me but turned away and didn't make an entry in the report book.

Sunday 29 March 1959

Vera Fish and Brian came to see me on his motor bike. Brian went off to the social centre while I took Vera round the grounds. When they had gone, I went off to see Ruthie Wilson and sat with her on the bench behind the tennis courts. She had brought her transistor radio so we listened to the pop songs of Buddy Holly singing *It Doesn't Matter any More*, Bobby Day with *Rockin' Robin* and The Platters with *The Great Pretender* – how appropriate. I had to get back by 6:00 PM when Sister Bartholomew came back on duty as I didn't want to get into trouble yet again.

Monday 30 March 1959

Wilkie came round and said I can have some walking sticks and get up for three-quarters of a day. As it is Easter Monday and visitors are allowed, Mum, Pop, Ginger and Uncle Eddie arrived. After they went Mickey Paris and Lulu popped in and I took them round the grounds. I tried to find Ruthie but she must have been on duty. That missing dressing gown was eventually found hanging behind a bathroom door – panic over.

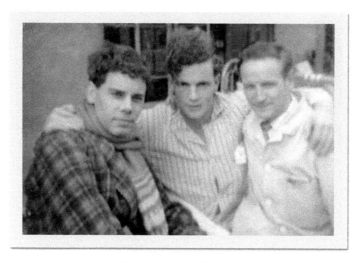

Me, Irish Michael Flaherty and Orderly Brian Hunnable.
Notice the scarf that I knitted from wool supplied by OT and Pop's
dressing gown that mysteriously disappeared then reappeared.

Tuesday 31 March 1959

Afternoon, went to the social centre with Bill Webb and Michael Foster.
Saw Ruthie there so I went off with her to the tennis courts. Arranged to
see her back there at 7:00 PM but she didn't turn up so I went back to the
ward. No *Rockin' Robin* today.

Wednesday 1 April 1959

Got up at 11:15 AM and went round the grounds with Peter Collinson.
Afternoon, Clifford Glascoe came to see me and we went for a walk. My
ankle is swelling up – must take it easy and not go out walking so much.
Might go for a ride in Clifford's car tomorrow if Sister gives permission.
Ruthie walked past the ward and gave me a cheery wave but the Matron
was watching. Ruthie might get into trouble; 'Fraternising with the
patients is not allowed' yeah, yeah. Received a card from Ron Jurgens,
art teacher at Tottenham County School.

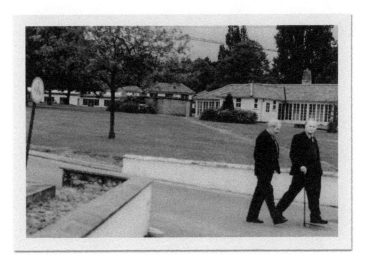

A more recent 1997 photo showing the wall in front of the social centre where we sat spending many happy hours watching the nurses go by.

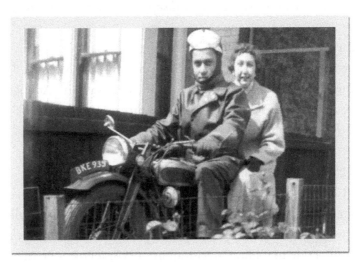

Brother Brian often visited me bringing a friend on the back of his motorbike. This bike is his 1934 Royal Enfield. His passenger is cousin Brenda but she did not come to the hospital.

Thursday 2 April 1959

Michael Foster came in with a black eye – he wouldn't say who did it. Serves the bugger right. Clifford Glascoe called for me at 2:30 PM and drove me to his Halifax Building Society office in Braintree to meet his staff then to his home. Met his wife Joan. It is very strange being back in a domestic house and seeing wallpaper again – it has been such a long time since I have seen any. He drove me back to the hospital at 6:00 PM. Messed round on the ward then to bed.

Friday 3 April 1959

Morning, went to the social centre. Afternoon, went for a stroll with Bill and Michael. Left them after a while and met Ruthie at 2:30 PM on the bench by the tennis courts – she went back to the nurses' home at 4:15 PM. Evening, phoned the nurses' home and arranged to meet Ruthie at 9:30 PM. After lights out I crept over the grass to Astins Ward but Ruthie wasn't there, so I crept back late and Italian orderly Tony helped me evade the duty nurse on night shift.

Saturday 4 April 1959

George Moase helped me get into a real bath – such luxury! Afternoon, went out with Irish Michael and Geoff Purl – sat on the wall outside the social centre and chatted to the nurses.

Sunday 5 April 1959

Morning, went to the social centre with Irish Michael. Afternoon, Mum, Pop and Ginger came to see me. Pop got permission from Sister to take me out in his car so we drove to Halstead and around the countryside. Very nice to get out of the grounds again, officially this time. Evening, all the patients got together on the ward and sang rock'n'roll songs to record on my Grundig.

Monday 6 April 1959

Wilkie did his rounds. Phoned Ruthie but we couldn't meet at the tennis courts due to heavy rain – rain stopped play. When it stopped, I sneaked out of the grounds to the village with Bill Webb then back to the social centre. In the evening I chatted with Charlie Squires and Michael Foster then went to bed.

Tuesday 7 April 1959

Felt lazy so stayed in bed all morning then went to the social centre with the blokes. Wandered round the grounds with Derek Gentry and Michael – two new patients.

Wednesday 8 April 1959

Afternoon, Alan came to see me. Wandered round the grounds with him and ended up in the social centre. We had supper in the day room. Was supposed to see Ruthie but it didn't work out.

Thursday 9 April 1959

Got up and went to the social centre. Afternoon, went out with Irish Michael but it rained so we went back and I wrote some letters. Evening, bunked over to Astins Ward and chatted a blonde nurse then Ruthie turned up, but I had to go because she was on duty.

Friday 10 April 1959

Wilkie and some other doctors came round and saw me in the treatment room. Afternoon, went out with Irish Michael and chatted to Nurses Eunice and Margaret. Evening, bunked out to phone Ruthie but a fat woman in the phone box wouldn't come out so I gave up and went back to the ward.

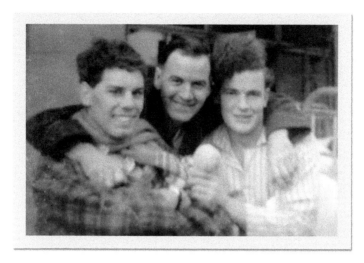

*Another two photos on the ward showing me with my knitted
bobble scarf and the dressing gown that caused so much grief.
Also shown are Bill Webb and Irish Michael Flaherty.*

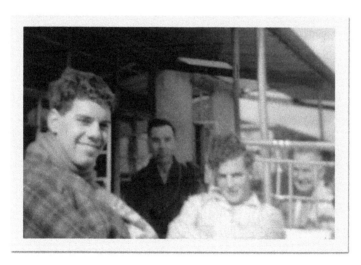

This picture also shows Dave Taylor, the chap on the extreme right.

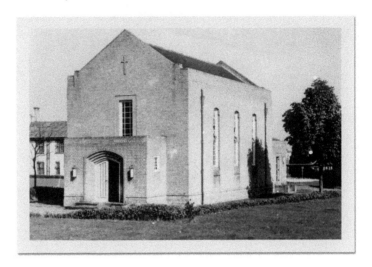

*The hospital Catholic Church where Wilkie often
conducted the services.*

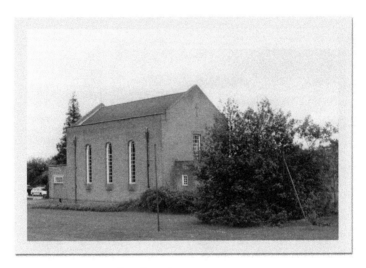

The same church taken during my return visit in 1997.

Saturday 11 April 1959

Orderly Italian Joe helped me take a bath. Feeling scrubbed up and confident I went to the nurses' home with Irish Michael and they let us into the lounge. Chatted to some nurses we hadn't seen before – Suzette Robinson and Irish Mary Boyle. They both turned up on the ward at 7:30 PM and asked us out. When things were quiet, Michael and I bunked out at 8:00 PM and met them at the tennis courts. We got back on the ward at 10:00 PM. Sister was on duty but we dodged her.[3]

Sunday 12 April 1959

Went to the Catholic Church in the grounds with Irish Michael to meet Nurses Mary Boyle and Suzette Robinson there. Wilkie conducted the service. Afterwards we went with Mary and Suzette to the social centre. Afternoon, Brian, Lulu and Mickey Paris came in. Took them out for a walk and left the grounds towards the village. Brian was worried I would get into trouble. Too late for that mate!

Monday 13 April 1959

Wilkie came round and discharged Bill Webb. Afternoon, I went to the social centre with Irish Michael and met nurses Margaret Lever and Valerie Hill. We arranged to take them to the social centre cinema next Thursday. Later on Bill Webb's family arrived in a car to take him home. Irish Michael and I met Mary Boyle and Suzette by the phone box and took them to the benches behind the tennis courts. Got back to the ward at 9:00 PM and sneaked in.

---

[3] After my discharge, Mary Boyle came to see me at home in Enfield.

Tuesday 14 April 1959

Bunked out of the grounds to the village with Irish Michael. On the way back we went to Ward 7 and chatted to Barbara in the laundry room and nurse Valerie Hill. We arranged to see them later but it suddenly stormed. When it stopped at 6:30 PM I went out and gave a note to Mary Boyle who was back on duty. Later I went to the nurses' home and chatted up some medical students in the training centre.

Wednesday 15 April 1959

Morning, went to the social centre with Michael Foster then over to see Reg Perkins who used to play cricket for Essex. I then went to J Ward to see Mavis – she had been moved there. We chatted until 5:00 PM. Got a letter from Mary Boyle asking me to go to the tennis courts after supper. I bunked out and waited on the bench but Mary didn't come – Valerie came instead. When Michael found out he had a go at me because he fancied Valerie so he went after Ruthie to get his own back. That bloke's a menace – don't trust him. Why can't he be content with just one nurse? Saw Hughie and the lads wandering around the grounds.

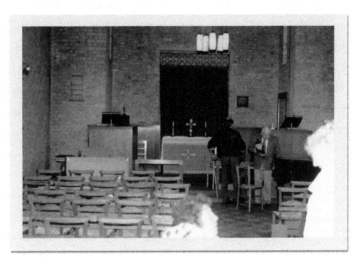

The interior of the Catholic Church taken during my 1997 visit.

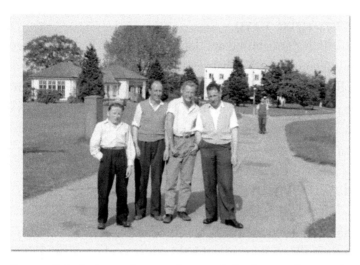

Some of the lads on the prowl around the hospital grounds.
Hughie Keating, Tom Rowley, David Evans and John Duffy.

Thursday 16 April 1959

Morning, met Valerie as arranged yesterday. Afternoon, went to the social centre cinema to see *The Last of the Mohicans*. Tried to sit with Nurse Margaret Lever but someone got there first. In the evening I sent a note to Nurse Mary Boyle suggesting we meet later today, then bunked out to J Ward to see Mavis. Left Mavis at 8:00 PM then went behind Ward 1 to meet Mary Boyle. Stayed with her until 10:00 PM then crept back to the ward. I saw Peter Collinson and Geoff Purl creeping back at the same time – I don't know what they had been up to. Unfortunately we were all missed by Staff Nurse Taffy who had sent out two orderlies looking for us. I told him I had just popped out to use the phone box. He didn't believe me and said he will report me to Wilkie.

Friday 17 April 1959

Staff Nurse Taffy came round and told me to stay in bed and not go out.
Wilkie didn't come but Miss Palmer the Deputy Matron came in and
told me off and reminded me that I must not fraternise with the nurses
or female patients. Why pick on me – Peter and Geoff were out as well?
Got up at 2:00 PM and sent a note to Nurse Mary Boyle telling her I have
been grounded again.

Saturday 18 April 1959

After the shift changed, I bunked out to the nurses' home and saw Mary
Boyle in their common room. Then suddenly the ward sisters arrived
including Sister Bartholomew so I hid in their washroom until the coast
was clear. Mary couldn't bunk out with me to Braintree so I went with
Barbara, a German trainee nurse who I chatted up on the bus. Went to
the bus park café with her and two other nurses came in – Susie and
Sylvia. I phoned Clifford Glascoe at the Halifax Building Society and he
joined us for tea. Got the bus back to the ward and made it just in time
before Staff Nurse Taffy came on duty. He never knew I had left the
ward let alone gone to Braintree on the bus.

Sunday 19 April 1959

Asked Staff Nurse Taffy if I could leave the ward to go to church –
he agreed as long as I come back straight after the service. Met
Mary Boyle outside the church and we went in together. Wilkie, who
was conducting the service, saw us but nothing was said afterwards.
Maybe he thought I was just being a good Catholic boy. In the afternoon
Mum, Pop, John, Alan, Mickey Paris, Joe Trow and Doreen all came to
see me. I didn't tell anyone what I had been up to. After lights out and
shift change, I popped over to see Mavis then met Mary Boyle behind
Ward 1 for an hour or so.

Monday 20 April 1959

Wilkie did his rounds – plaster can come off Thursday. Wandered round the grounds but nothing doing so went back to the ward then to see Mavis who is going home soon. Geoff Purl got a date with a blonde nurse from the kids' ward. I went out after lunch and chatted to Mary Boyle near the nurses' home but the Deputy Matron caught me and told me to go back to the ward, and she had a go at Mary for fraternising.

Tuesday 21 April 1959

We all got up early so they could move us from Denton Ward to Ward 1. Afternoon, Irish Michael went out with Nurse Diana Thomas so I went for a walk with Nurse Margaret Lever, keeping a watch out for Matron. Evening, went over to the tennis courts and watched the nurses playing tennis. Saw a nurse undressing behind a bush putting on her tennis gear. I found out later her name is Carmen from Spain. Wish I had my camera with me.

Wednesday 22 April 1959

Went outside to phone Clifford Glascoe. Afternoon, went back to the tennis courts again to watch the nurses playing tennis, and saw Mavis outside in a chair. Went out with the lads in the evening and chatted up Mary Boyle. Watched nurses playing ball behind Ward 1. Walking better now.

Thursday 23 April 1959

Wilkie came in and had a go at me for fraternising with the nurses – wonder who told him, or maybe he saw me in church with Nurse Mary Boyle. Went to the plaster room to have it removed – sheer luxury. Must use crutches for a week which buggered up my plan to take my mate John McEwan to the nurses' home. Evening, went out in a wheelchair with Michael and Geoff. Peter Collinson was down Snakey Lane with Nurse Carol. *"Now I know why they call it Snakey Lane"* she told me afterwards.

Friday 24 April 1959

Morning, went to the social centre on my crutches. In the afternoon I met Mary outside the ward and we went to Ward 7 where we chatted with nurses Janet, Elizabeth, Jocelyn, Carol and Lynn. They all had to go so I went back to the social centre and joined Irish Michael there. Evening, went out with Michael and saw Mary in the grounds. Chatted to her then the Deputy Matron suddenly appeared. She gave us another telling off and sent Mary back to the nurses' home. Evening, a new female nurse from Holland called Yoka arrived working nights. I had a recording session with the boys then Yoka borrowed my Grundig to play it in Sister's office. After lights out, I joined her in the office.

Saturday 25 April 1959

Morning, went to the phone box and 'tapped out' the Halifax Building Society in Edmonton and spoke to Pattie Lewis and Valerie Keig. Then Yoka and her friend came to my bed to listen to some of my recordings. John McEwan arrived at 2:30 PM. Weather was bad so we didn't go out. We had supper on the ward then he suggested that we bunk out to the village pub for a quick pint or two. Strictly forbidden of course but I sneaked out to phone Mr Duck who met us at the hospital entrance in his mini cab and drove us to The Vine pub. John and I each downed four pints in about an hour and I got back to the ward just in time for the 8 o'clock curfew. John went off home – both of us were a bit sloshed.[4]

---

[4] On another return visit to the hospital in October 2009, I measured the distance from the hospital main gate to The Vine pub – it is exactly half a mile. Add to this another 500 yards to the ward, which makes a total distance of three-quarters of a mile, each way. Well, Wilkie did tell me to get some exercise. I cannot understand why Mr Duck drove us to The Vine when another pub, The Reindeer, is much closer to the hospital.

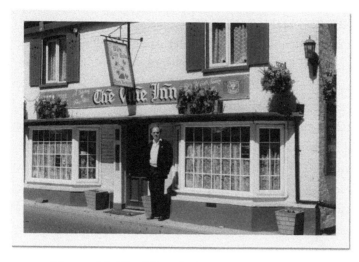

Me outside The Vine during my visit in 1997.

Sunday 26 April 1959

Mr Duck came round the ward with the morning papers but naturally said nothing about the visit to The Vine. Went to church then to the social centre with Mary, Susie and Sylvia. Afternoon, Brian, Ron and Maureen Copsey visited me. After they went I foolishly told some of the other blokes I had been down the pub yesterday so they all wanted to come. Word got round and by the time we had decided to bunk out after supper, half the ward joined us. So I took them out through the gate and invaded The Vine at about 7:00 PM. No mini cab this time – we got there on wheelchairs, crutches and sticks – it's a long way. We returned at 9:00 PM most of us drunk and some fell in the ditch near the entrance. The ward was in uproar. Sister had alerted security but cancelled it when we arrived. She went potty and sent us to bed saying we will be reported, naming me as ringleader. Why me – I am the youngest?

Monday 27 April 1959

Woke up with a terrible hangover. Sister came round still very angry and said Wilkie wants to see everyone who went to the pub. He had us in the office one by one – all the others got away with a warning but he threw the book at me when he found out I had been down the pub with John the day before and assumed I was the ringleader. He was really mad and said I will be discharged from hospital for *"behaviour inconsistent with hospital rules"*. Later on, when he had calmed down, he said he will let me off as long as I don't do anything like that again, but it had already been reported to the hospital committee. Maybe I had impressed Wilkie by going to his church but he didn't know I only went there to meet the nurses. The Sister tightened up on everything – we must all stay on the ward all day from now on. So in the evening I played housy-housy with the boys then went to sleep.

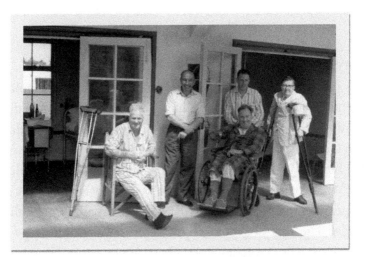

Some of the patients who came with me to The Vine.
Left to right standing: Reg Perkins, John Duffy and Orderly
Roy Gatwood who just happened to be there for the photo.
Left to right sitting: Wally Clarke and Ted Fryer.

Tuesday 28 April 1959

Morning, stayed on the ward and behaved myself. Afternoon, Sister was off duty so I asked Staff Nurse Taffy if I could go to the social centre to play billiards as recommended by physiotherapy as good exercise – that's what I told him anyway. He agreed because he hadn't yet caught up with the news about The Vine. I went out to the billiard hall and chatted a nurse there from Astins.

Wednesday 29 April 1959

Put 5 bob on a horse but it lost. Clifford Glascoe came into see me and later I went to the social centre where I met Nurse Valerie Hill. Arranged to meet tomorrow morning.

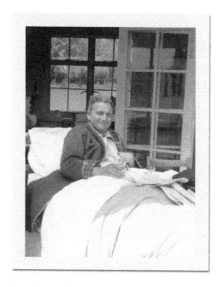

*Leslie Frostick – always warned me when
Sister was on the prowl. He used a mirror
to see through the rear window.*

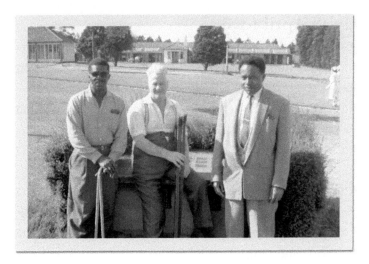

Left to right: Lionel Bryan, Wally Clarke and Eric Innes.
Lionel and Eric entertained us with their Negro Spirituals.

Thursday 30 April 1959

Morning, met Valerie and later we went to the social centre cinema.
Afterwards I recorded Lionel Bryan and Eric Innes singing Negro
spirituals including *A little more oil in my lamp keep me burning.*
Evening, went out with Geoff Purl for a stroll. Orderly Les Hackett
back on day duty.

Friday 1 May 1959

Morning, had a bath then sent birthday cards to John and Alan.
Afternoon, went to the social centre and saw Mavis in her wheelchair
with her two friends from the ward. Wandered off to the village with
Geoff – Michael was out with Nurse Margaret Lever. I received a parcel
of goodies from Boyka in Yugoslavia. Evening, went to the social centre
and chatted to Carmen, the Spanish nurse I saw undressing behind
a screen a few days ago. Italian orderly Tony tried to chat her but she
didn't want to know.

Saturday 2 May 1959

Books from Readers Digest arrived in the post. Sister Bartholomew came
in to tell me I might have to go in front of the hospital committee to be
disciplined about the pub visit. I thought I had squared that already with
Wilkie but it's up to the committee now. Geoff Purl, who was due to be
discharged anyway, was told to go at 1:30 PM – I don't know why, he has
been a bit naughty with the nurses and the pub visit but so have some of
the others. Anyway, I'll worry about that later – it's cup final day and the
McEwan twins' birthday so why worry about a committee? Went round
the grounds in the afternoon with Lionel Bryan and Eric Innes and
chatted with two nurses from Astins.

Sunday 3 May 1959

Morning, went to the Catholic Church to try and curry favour with
Wilkie. In the afternoon Mum, Pop and Ginger came in. After they left
I went out to see Mavis for a while. Evening, played solo with Dave and
Tom – lost 4/2d.

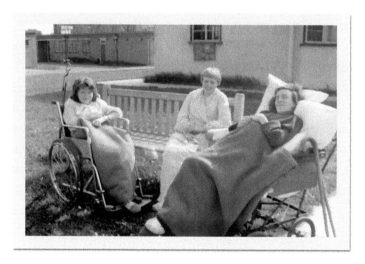

Mavis Peach (left) with her friends Sally and Janet Mayhew
enjoying a rare outing round the grounds.

Monday 4 May 1959

Wilkie came round and said he had already reported me to the committee even though I thought he had forgiven my sins. I decided I had better stay on the ward in case they summoned me. During the afternoon Wilkie came back and told me that I should be out in 2 — 3 weeks. At least I wasn't being chucked out like Geoff Purl. Later on Doctor 'Persian Pete' gave me a BSR whatever that is, then I went to bed and played my Grundig.

Tuesday 5 May 1959

Went to the social centre and chatted a Chinese nurse there. Later I went over to Ward J and with patients Sylvia and Sally, I pushed Mavis round the grounds in her wheelchair while Michael sneaked out to Braintree with Nurse Margaret Lever. Sister Bartholomew caught me with Mavis and sent me back to the ward. Later on the Deputy Matron arrived and took me into the office for a telling off again. Bloody hell, can't do anything in this place! Had a haircut by the visiting barber then played solo with Dave, Tom and Les Perkins. Evening, broke a tooth on a sausage then Sister came round for yet another nagging.

Wednesday 6 May 1959

Afternoon, Clifford Glascoe and an inspector from the Halifax Building Society visited me and discussed a possible convalescence in Switzerland, paid for by the Society. Best bit of news for ages.[5] After they went I sent a note over to Mavis. Michael bunked out with Nurse Margaret. Evening, stayed on the ward – no alternative as I must stay in after 4:30 PM as punishment.

---

[5]   However nothing came of Switzerland and I went to Deal instead – see Part 2.

Thursday 7 May 1959

Went over to OT with Reg Perkins and saw Hughie on the way back.
Met Irish Michael and we went to Cressing village with my camera and
met nurses Eunice Smith, Margaret Lever and Janet Baynham. Chatted
to the nurses then went back to the ward for my curfew at 4:30 PM.

Friday 8 May 1959

Sister is off duty – good. Went with Irish Michael to Cressing again. We
saw Wilkie drive past in his car but he didn't see us. Chatted to Valerie
Hill. Got back at 4:30 PM and played draughts with Dave.

Saturday 9 May 1959

Patient Alan Jones asked me, the next time I go to Braintree, to buy
a pair of black knickers with red cherries on them as a gift for his girl
friend Lucy. This time I asked Sister's permission to take the bus to
Braintree – she was in a good mood for a change and said I could go.
I found a women's shop and asked the assistant for black knickers with
cherries on but they only had plain black ones. I couldn't spend all
day looking round the shops so I bought those for 9/6d. Once outside,
a chap assumed I was a patient by my sticks and introduced himself as
Mr Boarder, the hospital administrator, and his wife. They wondered
what I had bought – I evaded the question. Mr Boarder was very friendly
and drove me to their home for tea then back to the ward at 7:00 PM,
clearing my late return with Sister. He also told me he is on the hospital
committee – now that could be handy.

Sunday 10 May 1959

Went to the Catholic Church then wandered round the grounds with Irish Michael. Brian and Vera visited me in the afternoon. Afterwards I popped over to see Mavis.

Monday 11 May 1959

So hot today that I asked the orderlies to push my bed outside in the sun. Wilkie came round and said I could go home next week – fantastic news! Afternoon, strolled round the grounds then to the dentist to have a tooth pulled out. Evening, played solo then went over to see Mavis. She had a go at me for seeing too much of Mary Boyle. She doesn't know about the others.

Tuesday 12 May 1959

Went over to OT to pay them off. Afternoon, went out with Irish Michael but I saw Ruthie so I left Michael and took her to Braintree without permission. Spotted Sister in her car near the market so Ruthie and I hid behind a vegetable stall until she drove off. Took Ruthie to a café and had a steak dinner for six bob each. First steak I've had for months.

Wednesday 13 May 1959

Morning, Irish Michael and Dave left the hospital and went home on a coach. Afternoon, Clifford Glascoe came in and we left the ward to chat on a bench. We then went to the social centre and said goodbye and I thanked him for visiting me so many times and being very kind. Evening, went to see Alan Jones whose girl friend Lucy was pleased with the black knickers I bought in Braintree – she didn't seem worried about the missing cherries. I asked her to put them on and show me but she just giggled.

Thursday 14 May 1959

Ted Fryer, Wally Clarke and John Duffy came into my room to have a chat. They went to the social centre cinema and I went to Cressing to take some photos. Saw Paul Griffiths there who works in the General Office with Sister. I asked him if he knew anything about me being called before the committee. He said the case has been dropped on the recommendation of Mr Boarder because I was going home soon anyway – nice to have influential contacts. Evening, went to the social centre then back to the ward. Chatted to Nurse Christine Reynolds. Turned on the Grundig but something happened and it went pop and blew the fuses in the ward. An electrician was called who soon fixed it. Slept outside as it is a warm night.

Friday 15 May 1959

Morning, went to the social centre to get some stuff for the boys. A few new patients were admitted to the ward – they will soon learn the ropes. Afternoon, Reg Perkins took me to Braintree in his car. Popped into the Halifax Building Society branch to see Clifford Glascoe. Met Reg's wife and kids and had tea with them. They took me back to the hospital in the car. Chatted to Yoka then went over to see Mavis. I don't sneak around any more, I'm demob happy!

Saturday 16 May 1959

Again, went to the social centre shop to buy some more things for the boys. Afternoon, went to the village then to Cressing Station. Another bloke from the committee saw me and gave me a lift back. Evening, went over to see Mavis and took a photo of her.

Sunday 17 May 1959

Morning, went to church. In the afternoon Mum, Pop and Ginger came in but as I didn't expect them, I was out round the grounds chatting to nurses Jane and Janet Warner. They found me eventually.

Monday 18 May 1959

Saw Wilkie in the day room and he discharged me. Phoned Blondie (a neighbour) asking her to tell Mum the news so I can be collected tomorrow. Went to the nurses' home and round the grounds to tell all the nurses and other staff that I will go tomorrow. Went over to see Mavis and made a note of her home address. We were then told that the whole ward is moving to Ward 8, back to where I started months ago. Wonder if the bats are still there.

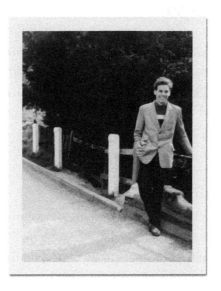

A photo of me when I bunked out to
Cressing, taken by Nurse Margaret Lever.
My sticks are out of range of the camera.

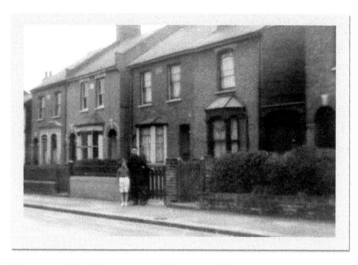

Sister and brother waiting for me at home in Putney Road,
Enfield. Notice the absence of cars at the time.

Tuesday 19 May 1959

During the morning we all moved back to Ward 8 – the circle is
complete. I was admitted there 280 days ago on 12 August 1958 before
being moved to Denton Ward. Didn't see any bats this time. Said
cheerio to all patients and staff. Sister Bartholomew even gave me a hug
before she told me that I was a troublesome patient but brought a ray of
sunshine to the hospital – how nice. I also went to find the contrite Jim
Brown and shook his hand to show there are no hard feelings. He was
very relieved at the gesture. Mum and Pop arrived and loaded me and
my stuff into the car, and we left the hospital and drove home.

Home at last but in the evening, feeling unsettled, I took a bus to
Waltham Cross to see Maureen Copsey and her family, then phoned
Vera Fish. I took the bus back and saw Mum and Pop looking for me
round the top of the road wondering where I had got to.

I cannot forget Black Notley Hospital and the kindness and care provided by the staff. In the intervening period of six weeks before convalescence I returned there to see the nurses and any remaining patients.

After adjusting to family and social life I was sent to a convalescent home in Deal, Kent for a further period of rest. However my time there turned out to be rather less restful than intended – see Part 2.

PART 2

THE ROAD TO RECOVERY

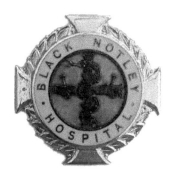

Saturday 4 July 1959

John came round at 12 o'clock and joined Mum and Pop driving me to Charing Cross Station. Once on the train I met Ted Peggs and Pete Green, also going to Caxton Memorial Home in Deal. Ted is on crutches after an accident. When we arrived I registered at the home, read the rule book then had dinner. Afterwards Ted and I went to a nearby pub to get acquainted. When we got back to Caxton the front door was locked – we had forgotten about the 10:00 PM curfew from the rule book. So we crept round the back, found an open door and bunked in before the night porter did his rounds and locked up.

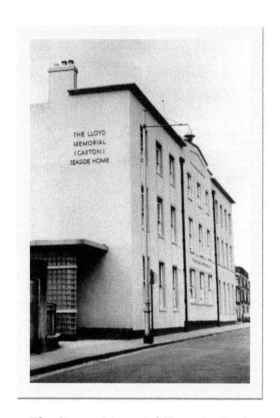

The Caxton Memorial Home in Deal.
Postcard: © D V Bennett Ltd, Maidstone.

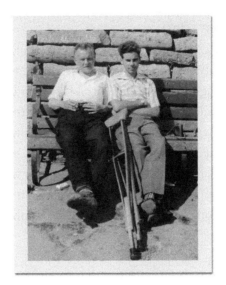

*Ted and I near Deal relaxing
in the sun. The crutches are Ted's.*

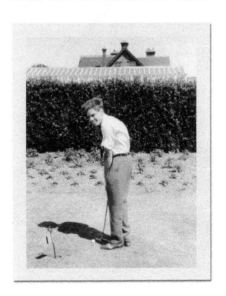

Putting Green in Walmer.

Sunday 5 July 1959

Had breakfast then lounged around wondering how to spend our time there. In the afternoon I pushed Ted around town in a wheelchair borrowed from Caxton. Later that evening we wandered around Deal and found the Oasis Club where got free membership for a month.

Monday 6 July 1959

Went to Walmer with Ted and Pete and had a game on the putting green. We popped into the Conservative Club and showed my membership card, so they let us in. Had lunch in Walmer, returned to Caxton for dinner then went down the pub.

Tuesday 7 July 1959

Went round the shops in Deal with Ted and Pete. We bought some fishing tackle and hired a boat for three hours – caught a big fish. I pulled in the anchor and nearly fell in the water.

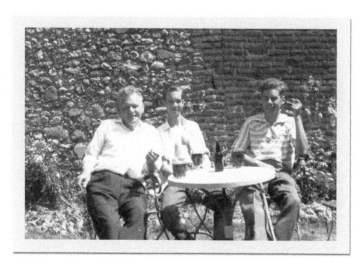

What did my doctor say about the booze?

Wednesday 8 July 1959

Took a bus to Kingsdown to see friends of Ted's in the post office. After lunch we lazed around on the beach. Back in Deal we had dinner at Caxton then tried a couple of the local pubs.

Thursday 9 July 1959

After a lazy morning we went on the pier for some fishing but caught nothing. We chatted up three girls on the pier who told us they were musicians booked to play as a trio that evening (cello, violin and piano) at the Quarterdeck Theatre. They invited us to their concert and we agreed to go. In the afternoon we went to the small shop opposite Caxton and met the owner Mrs Anderson. She said business is slow so I suggested she could clear some space in the shop and sell tea and cakes to the inmates of Caxton. We offered to help organise it and get customers. After dinner we went to the Quarterdeck to hear the trio. It finished after curfew but I saw the town mayor in the audience wearing his chains so I cheekily asked him if he could get us back into Caxton. He drove us there in the limo and got us past the night porter.

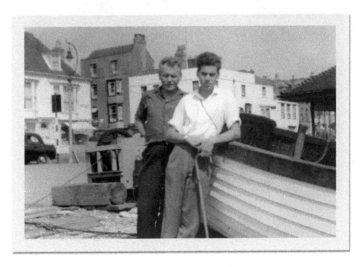

Fishing trip near Deal pier.

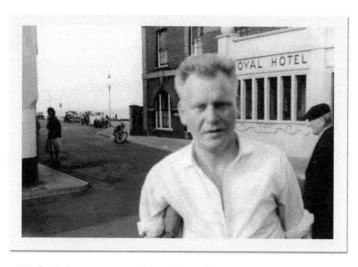

With Ted we went to the pub to discuss our new venture.

Friday 10 July 1959

In the morning Ted and I popped over to see Mrs A and planned our tea shop. We then went back to Caxton and scrounged some cups, saucers and spoons for her shop so she could sell teas. Then we went to the bar at the Royal Hotel to discuss our new venture.

Saturday 11 July 1959

Morning, went round the shops and had lunch in Cathy's Café. Later we went to a garden fete then round the town in the evening. We returned to Caxton after the curfew so bribed the night porter with two shillings to let us in.

Sunday 12 July 1959

We took some inmates from Caxton over to Mrs A's tea shop – her first customers. She is very happy. During the afternoon we went for a walk on the pier. After dinner we went down the pub but got back late again, bribing the night porter with two bob to let us in.

Monday 13 July 1959

Went to Canterbury for the day; did some shopping, visited the cathedral then popped into the Halifax Building Society branch to withdraw some cash. Back at Caxton we had dinner then went to the Oasis Club. Again we bribed the night porter to let us in.

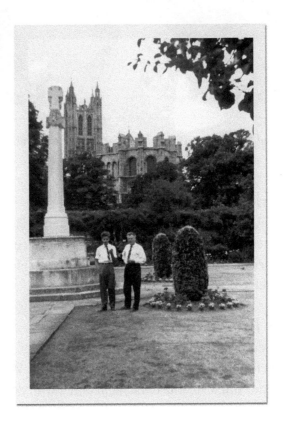

Ted and I on a day trip to Canterbury.

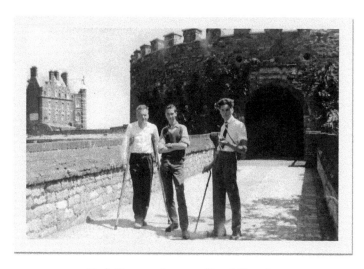

Ted, Pete and me at Deal Castle.

Tuesday 14 July 1959

Took a bus to Sandwich and went fishing on the river. Caught nothing but a bloke there caught an eel and gave it to us. We took it back to Caxton and gave it to the cook. Went to the Oasis Club again. Back late – another two bob.

Wednesday 15 July 1959

Went round the shops and had lunch. In the evening we missed dinner in Caxton so we went to the Oasis Club instead. Tried their vintage cider and got back late again at 11:30 PM feeling sick – must be the cider. Had to bribe the porter again to get back in.

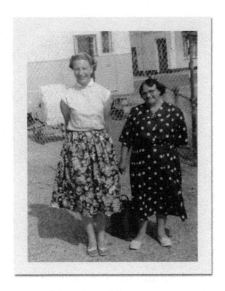

Mary Brown and her friend Lou Davey arrive at Deal.

Thursday 16 July 1959

Bought a fresh chicken in a butchers for ten shillings and some
vegetables from a greengrocer. In the evening we took our purchases to
Mrs A's shop. She cooked the chicken and veg and we all had a meal in
her tea room.

Friday 17 July 1959

Spent the day cleaning Mrs A's shop ready for more customers. Went
boozing after dinner at Caxton.

Saturday 18 July 1959

New arrivals at Caxton – Mary Brown with her older friend Louise
Davey, both from North Kensington. Chatted up Mary and went for
a walk with her to Kingsdown.

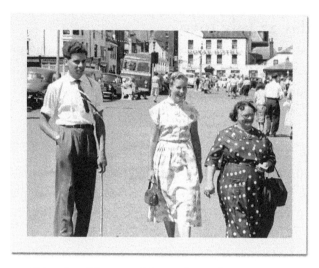

Showing Mary and Lou where the action is.

Sunday 19 July 1959

Spent most of the day walking around Deal with Mary and Lou –
showing them where to go and the nightlife.

Monday 20 July 1959

Mary is getting very friendly. Afternoon, went to Mrs A's shop with Ted
to fix her blind then to the Oasis Club in the evening where we spent all
our money – had nothing left to bribe the night porter so we went round
Mrs A's shop and she let us in at 11 o'clock. Ted slept in the spare bed
upstairs and I crashed out in the armchair downstairs. Ted complained
he was bitten by fleas all night.

Tuesday 21 July 1959

Went to the bank to get some cash. Bought some crabs and ate them on
the beach. Oasis Club in the evening.

Wednesday 22 July 1959

Saw Ted off at the station who went back to London for a hospital check-up. Went round the shops with a rich bloke staying at Caxton. Afternoon, walked to Sandwich Bay with Mary and later, took her and Lou to the Oasis Club.

Thursday 23 July 1959

Went round the shops with Mary, Lou and Ella, another inmate at Caxton. Took Mary to the pictures to see *Fantasia*. Later we played bowls in the Caxton garden.

Friday 24 July 1959

Went to see Mrs A – her fridge is busted so I phoned the fridge people to come and fix it. Went to the station and met Ted back from London; now on two sticks instead of crutches. Took a taxi back to Caxton. Went for a stroll around Deal and Walmer with Mary, returning to Caxton late evening. It was pouring with rain so we sat in a bus shelter and fell asleep. We both woke up after curfew. We had no money to bribe the porter so we kipped in the bus shelter all night.

Saturday 25 July 1959

Mooched around all day, went to the bank then the Oasis Club with Ted, Mary and Lou. Ted bought some cigars – made me feel sick.

Sunday 26 July 1959

Ted's leg playing up so we went to see Matron who gave him some pills. Afternoon, went to Margate fairground with Ted. Bloke there had a flea circus. He offered a quid for a dozen fleas as he said they are difficult to find. We told him we know a place where there are fleas and asked him how to catch them. He said use cotton wool – the fleas jump in, get their legs caught and can't get out. He gave us his phone number. More bribes to get back into Caxton.

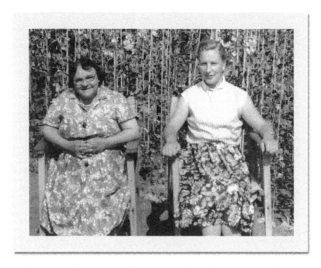

Lou and Mary relaxing in the Caxton garden.

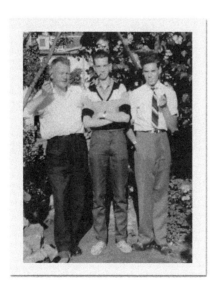

Ted, Pete and me in the Caxton garden.

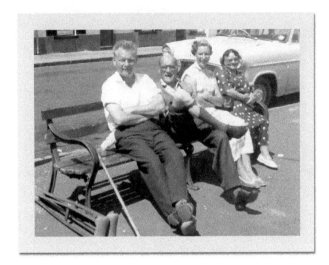

Ted, Charlie, Mary and Lou
on the sea front at Deal.

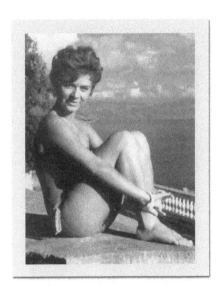

This is Boyka again. She had nothing
to do with Deal but is better looking
than the rest of us.

Monday 27 July 1959

Went round Mrs A's and told her we could get rid of her fleas. I scrounged some cotton wool and a jam jar from Caxton and went to work in Mrs A's spare room. We caught dozens of fleas in the cotton wool and put them in the jam jar. Went back to Caxton for a shower – we were lousy with them. Phoned the bloke at Margate who said he would come and collect them and pay us. Waited in all day but he didn't turn up, so we took them outside and let them loose. Evening, went to the Oasis Club and met Louie there who took me and Mary for a ride in his van. Got back to Caxton at midnight. Another two bob to get in.

Tuesday 28 July 1959

Intended going cockling but it started to rain so we went to Mrs A's shop. Evening, went to the Oasis Club then back to Mrs A's who cooked us a steak dinner.

Wednesday 29 July 1959

Went to Ramsgate to try cockling but it was raining too much. Wandered round the shops again and ended up in the Oasis Club.

Thursday 30 July 1959

Intended going to Hastings but decided it was too far. Afternoon, went to the Mariners Fete and had a good laugh. Planned a quiet evening at Caxton but went instead to the Oasis Club. Returned at 11:45 PM. Cost us more money to get back in.

Friday 31 July 1959

Not a lot – spent the morning at Caxton relaxing in the garden. Tried watering the plants but the hose broke and ended up spraying the other inmates. They were cross with me. Evening at the Oasis Club then late back to Caxton.

Saturday 1 August 1959

My birthday – 20 years old today! Time to go home. Said goodbye to
everyone and took the train to Charing Cross. Pop and Brian met me
at the station.

Got home at noon – Alan came round and we went to Enfield Town
library, met John there. Evening, went to an off-licence and bought
booze and cigars. Had a few beers in the Prince Albert then went round
the McEwan's place for a birthday booze up until midnight.

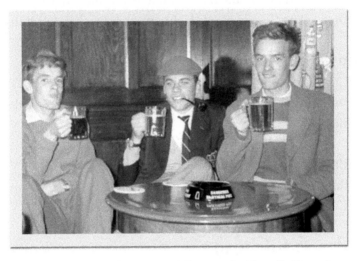

*A few pints in the Prince Albert with Alan (left) and
John (right) for my birthday.*

Recuperating in a country retreat

Together with the McEwan twins I enjoyed many restful weekend visits staying in their aunt's caravan in Danbury, Essex. At the time John was working at the Medical Research Council Labs in Carshalton while Alan was still at Hull.

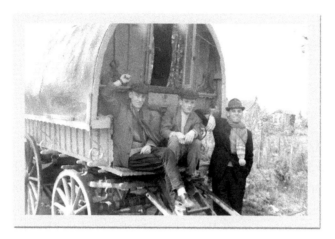

Aunt Lill's caravan on her farm in Danbury, Essex.

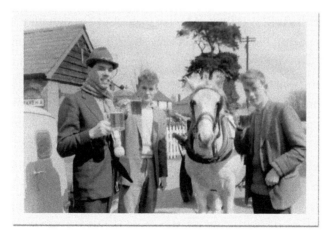

Daisy the horse pulled us in the cart to the local pub and back.

On 24 October, John and I paid a visit to Black Notley Hospital to wander the grounds and pop into the nurses' home. There we bumped into Valerie Hill and Mary Boyle. Leaving them to work their shift, we returned to the caravan in Danbury.

On 11 December we took Daisy the horse to the blacksmiths. Next day we left the caravan and went to Braintree for lunch with Clifford Glascoe then to the nurses' home where we met Christine Reynolds and Janet Baynham. When we left them it was late so we stayed the night in The Reindeer Pub, Black Notley.

Escape to Scandinavia

The Halifax Building Society was very good to me by paying my full wages for six months while I was in hospital, then half wages until I returned to work. When I did return, after convalescing in Deal, the Society allowed me to work short time on full pay for a further period. However, after a year I became restless and felt there is more to life than working in an office, especially after having spent a large chunk of my formative years in hospital. By chance I was invited to live in central Sweden for a while and it was an opportunity that I couldn't resist. So I spoke to the manager of the Society who understood my need to escape and see a bit of the world before settling down.

I was conscious that only 18 months previously I was lying in bed covered in plaster while harbouring fears that my future activities will be severely curtailed. But thanks to the skill of the surgeon and the nursing staff I now felt able to travel, work and find independence in a foreign land.

It was on 28 August 1960 that I packed my rucksack and took a coach to Newcastle and a boat to Oslo where I stayed for a few days. From Oslo I hitch-hiked north to Trondheim then took a train across the border to Hallen in Sweden. Once there I stayed with a family for several weeks trying to learn their language while working on their strawberry farm. I learnt to drive there – at the time Sweden drove on the left while Norway drove on the right.

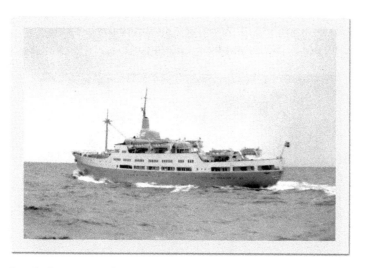

I sailed away on the MS Blenheim from Newcastle to Oslo.
(I took this photo from the deck of its sister ship, the MS Braemar,
during my return. The Christmas tree destined for Trafalgar Square
as an annual gift from Norway to England lay on the deck.)

After a few weeks living in Sweden I hitch-hiked back to Oslo but realised I hadn't enough money to return home so I found a job working in a large downstairs kitchen at the famous Metropol Restaurant and Jazz Club. I worked there often on double shift (16 hours a day) for six weeks and picked up quite a lot of the language.

From the kitchen I could hear the jazz bands upstairs but didn't know at the time that some of the most famous musicians in the world were performing there. These included Coleman Hawkins, Bud Powell, Stan Getz and more jazz luminaries now documented in the publication "*Born Under the Sign of Jazz*" by Randi Hultin.

I eventually saved enough money to return home by Christmas but exactly two years later my feet started itching again and I returned to Norway, but this time with John and Alan McEwan. We hitched from Enfield to Aberdeen, scrounged lifts in boats to the Shetlands, the Faeroes and onto Norway ending up working back at the Metropol.

Wilkie would certainly not have approved!

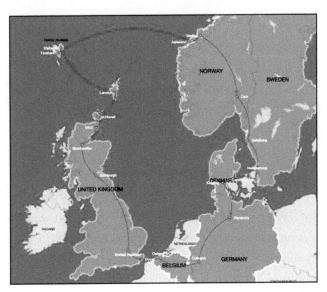

The second six-week Nordic adventure took us to the Shetlands, Faeroes, Norway and home via Sweden, Denmark, Holland, Germany and Belgium.

PART 3

RETURN VISITS

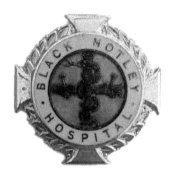

Fete and Funday at Black Notley Hospital

On 1 June 1997 I went to an open day at the hospital before it surrendered to a housing estate a year later. Central to the celebrations was the *Great Hip & Knee Walk* to raise money for the Wishbone Trust, a charitable organisation supporting research into joint and bone diseases. Here is the front cover of the programme of events, opened by Jimmy Greaves, former England footballer, TV sports commentator and presenter.

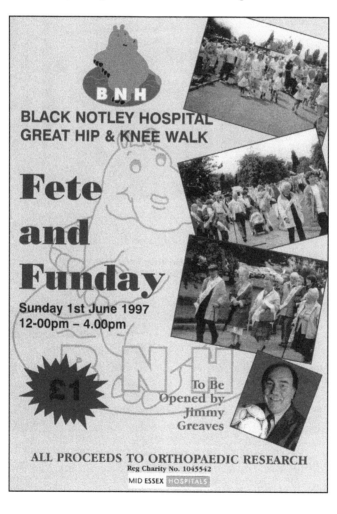

Return Visit in 1997

A month prior the Fete and Funday I joined a group of former patients and staff for a nostalgic visit to the hospital before it closed. The visit was organised by former patient Allen Jones who had spent 3.5 years in the hospital during the 1940s.

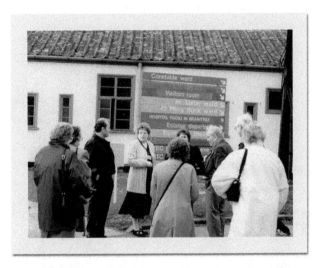

Allen Jones (third from left) is discussing the site plan and ward names with the group.

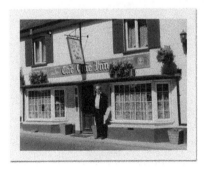

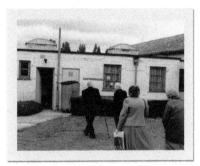

We had lunch in The Vine pub – my first official visit since 26 April 1959!

Checking out another building.

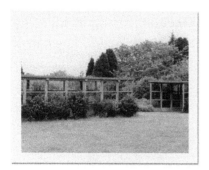

*The covered walkway allowing
access to some of the wards
when it rained.*

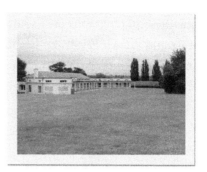

*Another view across the hospital
grounds showing the vast
expanse of lawn areas.*

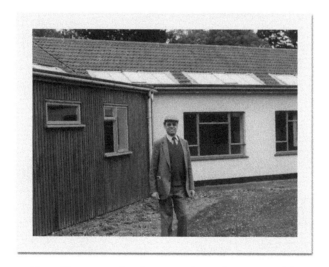

Standing outside what may have been Ward 8.

Return Visit in 2009

I took these photographs on 7 October 2009 during a visit with my wife Carole and the McEwans to the Braintree Museum. We had lunch in The Vine pub then visited the housing estate which is now on the site of the hospital.

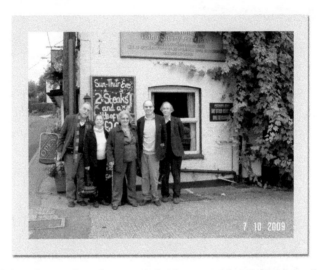

John, Betty, Carole, me and Alan outside The Vine pub.

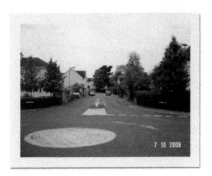

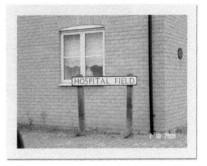

Main entrance to the housing estate built on the hospital site.

A reminder that the housing estate was once a hospital.

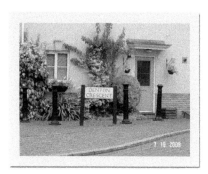

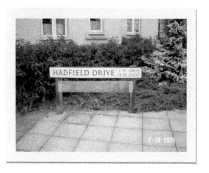

Even one of my wards is mentioned here.

A tribute to the hospital secretary Arthur Hadfield.

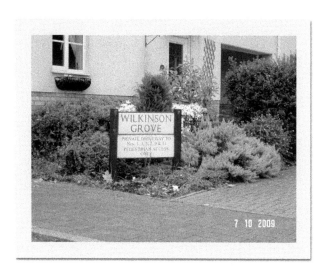

And a tribute to Mr Michael Wilkinson, Medical Superintendent and Orthopaedic Surgeon.

ACKNOWLEDGEMENTS

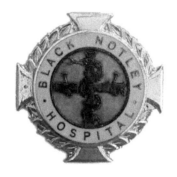

ACKNOWLEDGEMENTS

I want to pay tribute to the many people who took the trouble to come and see me – it was always a moment of pleasurable anticipation to tidy up the bed and side cabinet while the staff prepared the ward for the incoming visitors. They were generally allowed in each Sunday and Wednesday afternoons, although other days were possible. I rarely knew in advance who would walk through the door invariably bringing some goodies such as chocolates, smarties, beer and reading material.

It was not until my return visit to Black Notley that I realised how difficult it was for friends and family to visit me. The abundance of private cars around today makes the journey much easier but back in 1958-59 not everyone had a car and public transport was the only option. The exception to this was with the McEwan twins whose right thumbs were used to great effect in getting free transport.

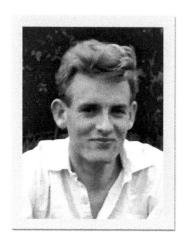 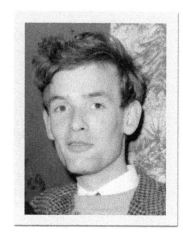

Alan McEwan   John McEwan

For a year or so after leaving hospital I was in touch with several patients and staff but eventually we drifted apart.

MR WILKINSON: on 12 November 1959 I attended a clinic at Wansted Hospital for an appointment with Wilkie and while there I was reunited with several former patients. He died in October 1980 after moving to the Isle of Man.

CLIFFORD GLASCOE: he moved to Wales to take up a position as branch manager and while there I popped in to see him while on holiday. In the seventies Clifford was promoted to area manager and he was responsible for getting me my first mortgage with the Halifax Building Society during a period when lending was at its lowest. Until I eventually lost touch with him, I sent Clifford and his wife Joan a box of Balkan Sobranie Cocktail cigarettes each Christmas.

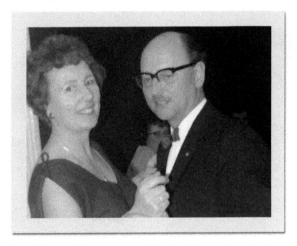

Clifford and Joan Glascoe at a Society dance in the '50s or '60s.
Photo: Courtesy of the Glascoe family.

BILL (STUBBY) LAGDON: I went to his home in Dagenham but he was out and have since heard nothing from him.

MAVIS PEACH: a patient and special friend but I lost touch with her soon after leaving hospital. She gave me her address in Porthill, Newcastle-under-Lyme, Staffordshire but didn't respond to my letters. I suspect that due to her very serious illness she may not have survived.

BILL WEBB: I wrote to him some years later but a letter came back from his brother-in-law telling me that Bill had died soon after leaving hospital.

NURSE MARY BOYLE: visited me at home in Enfield shortly after I was discharged but then we lost contact.

NURSE RUTHIE WILSON: tried to find her back at the hospital but she was on duty. Tried again but eventually lost touch.

Here is a list of my visitors – I am indebted to all of them. Some of their photos are on previous pages and continue on the following pages:

Mum, Pop, sister Susan (Ginger)
Uncles Eddie, Dave, Les, Fred and Tug Wilson
Alan and John McEwan
Mr and Mrs Trow
Brothers Brian and Ron
Alan (Joe) Trow, Doreen Picking
Tex (dog)
Ann Cawthorne, Vera Fish
Violet Phinn, Sid (SAJ) Brown
Clifford Glascoe
Maureen Copsey
Mickey Paris, Pam (Lulu) Butcher
Gary Wooding.

More of my visitors …

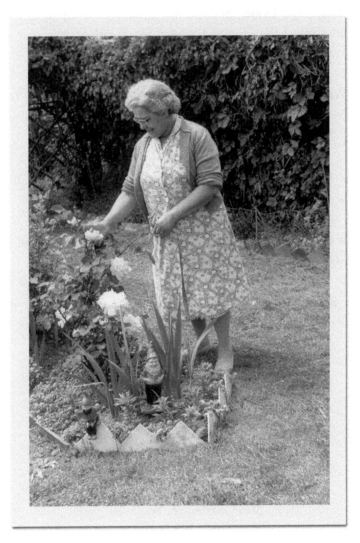

My mum, Elvina

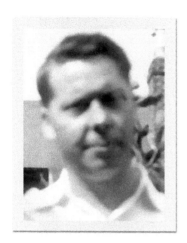

My dad, Bill

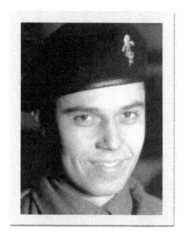

Brother Brian

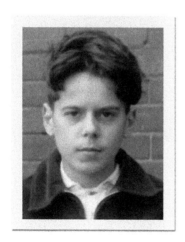

Brother Ron

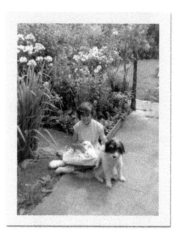

Sister Susan (Ginger)

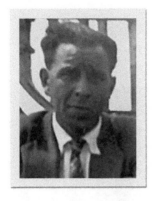

Uncle Eddie Paterson

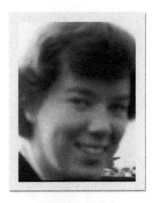

Vera Fish

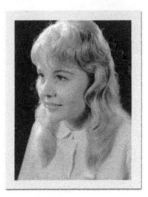

Maureen Copsey

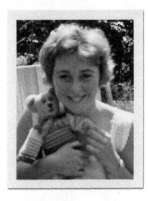

Pam (Lulu) Butcher

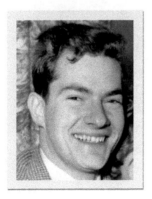

Mickey Paris

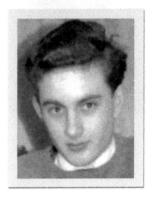

Alan (Joe) Trow

And what became of?

TED PEGGS at Deal: went to his house in Islington with John to buy his amplifier. Ted visited me then we lost contact.

MARY BROWN: continued seeing her for a year or more before I was invited to work in Scandinavia.

GRUNDIG TAPE RECORDER: used it until the mid '80s when the tape of the *Black Notley Blues* play and carol singers got screwed up in the mechanism and was beyond repair.

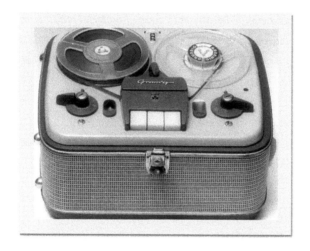

During the preparation of this book, many people have given generously with their time, wisdom and experience, and I am grateful to them. Special thanks are due to Dr Carole Reeves for agreeing to write the Foreword – without her advice and encouragement the book may never have been published. Particular mention also goes to Brian Jarvis on his invaluable editorial advice and assistance and the Braintree District Museum Trust Ltd for their kind cooperation in supplying the credited photographs.

Information Page

The author, Chris Dell, may be contacted via the publisher at
www.stortdoc.com

Other links:

Braintree District Museum Trust Ltd. www.braintreemuseum.co.uk.
*The Trust holds a comprehensive collection of material relating to the
Black Notley Hospital, consisting primarily of photographs, whilst the
Museum shop is stocked with local history publications, historical gifts,
postcards and photographic prints.*

Black Notley Community Association. www.thebnca.co.uk.
*The current premises are original existing features of the old Black Notley
Hospital that was demolished in 1998.*

Suggested reading:

Shaw, A., and C. Reeves. *The Children of Craig-y-nos: Life in a Welsh
Tuberculosis Sanatorium, 1922—1959.* London: Wellcome Trust Centre
for the History of Medicine at UCL, 2009 [ISBN 978-0-85484-126-4]

Wood, A., comp. *Black Notley Hospital: A Century of Service.*
Essex: Black Notley Parish Council, 1998. [ISBN 978-0-95334-020-0]
(This book is available from the Parish Clerk at info@blacknotley-pc.gov.uk)

Lightning Source UK Ltd.
Milton Keynes UK
UKHW02f1357260418
321614UK00005B/263/P